FEELING GOOD IS GOOD FOR YOU

CARL J. CHARNETSKI & FRANCIS X. BRENNAN

RODALE

Back cover photographs © by (from top to bottom) The Stock Market, Mel Curtis/PhotoDisc, Nina Rizzo/Stone, Luc Hautecoeur/Stone

Author photograph © Kurt Wilson

Printed in the United States of America

Rodale Inc. makes every effort to use acid-free (∞), recycled paper ♲ .

Cover and Interior Designer: Joanna Williams

The figures in the Rahe Life Stress Scale on page 76 are from *Journal of Psychosomatic Research* 43, Mark A. Miller and Richard H. Rahe, "Life Changes: Scaling for the 1990s," 1997, with permission from Elsevier Science.

The Pet Attitude Scale on page 130 is reprinted from *Psychological Record* 31, no. 3, Donald I. Templer, David M. Veleber, Charles A. Salter, Sarah Dickey, and Roy Baldwin, "The Construction of a Pet Attitude Scale," 1981, with permission.

Library of Congress Cataloging-in-Publication Data

Charnetski, Carl J.
    Feeling good is good for you : how pleasure can boost your immune system and lengthen your life / Carl J. Charnetski and Francis X. Brennan.
       p.   cm.
    Includes bibliographical references and index.
    ISBN 1–57954–346–4 hardcover
    1. Natural immunity.   2. Pleasure—Physiological aspects.
    3. Psychoneuroimmunology.   4. Natural immunity—Effect of stress on.
    I. Brennan, Francis X.   II. Title.
    QR185.2 .C475   2001
    616.07'9—dc21   2001002096

Distributed to the book trade by St. Martin's Press

2   4   6   8   10   9   7   5   3   1   hardcover

Visit us on the Web at www.rodalestore.com, or call us toll-free at (800) 848-4735.

Contents

Acknowledgments

With a project of this magnitude, there are many people to thank. We would first like to thank Nancy Hancock, our editor at Rodale, for her intellect, assistance, time, and patience over the last year.

We would like to thank Rodale Books vice president and publisher Neil Wertheimer, whose insight, judgment, and stewardship, along with Nancy's, helped make this book a reality.

We would also like to thank Lisa Andruscavage and her copy editors, who have been invaluable in translating our words from academese into English.

Margie Price typed most of the manuscript; not only is she incredibly facile with a word processor, but her very presence boosted our immunity during the long writing process. Sue Paoletti also typed portions of the manuscript and was generally a great help.

We must commend the hundreds of students at Wilkes University who consented to spit into cups for a few extra-credit points. Numerous other students helped us collect and analyze data, and we are very thankful to them. Thanks also to the faculty and administrative colleagues who helped and encouraged us. A special acknowledgment goes to reference librarian Brian Sacolic.

Thank you to the in-laws—Harry, Esther, Kathy, Ward, Cindy, Billy, Sally, and Eric—and their respective families. They have been a constant source of immunity-enhancing pleasure throughout the writing of this book.

Thank you to Bill and Ellie, and Jim and Charlotte, whose friendship and support has been invaluable. Thanks to fishing buddies Bob and Tony, who demanded a thorough and exacting scientific presentation of ideas related to the book before they considered them credible. Each fishing trip resulted in an oral defense of one part of our thesis, but it was a pleasure.

Thanks also to Dr. Georges M. Halpern for his information and inspiration.

Finally, we would like to thank our wives, Susan and Tina, for their patience and support. We spent many nights and weekends in front of the computer or reading, or both, and their love and understanding were essential.

Preface

All healing is self-healing.
—Albert Schweitzer, philosopher, music scholar, and missionary physician

Do you have aching arthritis? Is work often a stressful exercise in patience? Are you overweight? Do depressing thoughts darken your disposition? Are you prone to colds and the flu? Do you have a family history of heart disease or cancer? Are you, in short, worried about preserving good health or hastening the healing process?

If so, we have a specific formula for you to follow.

Don't worry—we're not going to demand that you embark on an exhausting exercise regimen, follow a strict, detailed diet, or expose yourself to a battery of invasive medical tests and procedures. Rather, we are proposing an adjunct therapy in which you drink a glass of fine wine, pet a cat or dog, make love to your mate, listen to some great music, and watch something funny on TV.

Why? Because each of these directives—from scratching your dog's belly to laughing at Jim Carrey's manic antics to hearing a beloved song to touching your partner—has been associated with strengthening of the immune system, your body's internal defense mechanism against infection, sickness, and disease.

And precisely what is the common denominator behind all of these feel-good prescriptions?

Pleasure.

Although the findings are relatively new—some documented just within the past decade or so and some not yet even published—the science behind them is solid and the evidence is sufficient to convince us that there is a critical connection between the mind's perception of pleasure and the body's ability to fend off illness.

Pleasure Principles, Principal Pleasures

Because of an ever-expanding body of medical and psychological knowledge, science is gaining insight into the delicate, complex interplays among the brain, the nervous system, and the immune system. Most of the literature in this burgeoning field has addressed the negative influences of stress, depression, and other psychological variables on immunological strength. But some researchers, ourselves included, have chosen to approach the issue from the other side of the coin, looking for positive ways to manipulate immune power to better prevent illness and more quickly restore health.

Plenty of research, including our own, now supports the contention that achieving and maintaining good health should not be a struggle, but a pleasure.

We know what you're thinking: How can you be happy and optimistic or have fun if you're sick? We won't argue this point. It is difficult to enjoy yourself when you are not feeling well. But science can now say with a good degree of certainty that if you are already ill, you have a much better chance of getting better, sooner, if you try to enjoy life and minimize stress and negativity. And if you aren't sick, you have a better chance of remaining well if you make pleasure a priority in your life.

In-Your-Head Medicine

It may seem trite, but to a great extent, illnesses of many sorts may indeed be in your head. This doesn't mean that you're crazy, but that you quite literally can think yourself into an ailment. If you believe you will get sick, a number of studies demonstrate that you very well may develop the symptoms that you anticipated. For instance, nausea is a common side effect of chemotherapy. Regularly treated cancer patients often start to get sick to their stomachs as soon as they pass through the doors of the oncology center.

Conversely, the exciting news is that much of medicinal healing is directly attributable not to some fabulous pharmaceutical or surgical procedure but to the simple power of mind over whatever matters to you. These estimations come not from advocates of alternative procedures or quacks; they come directly from a mountain of research amassed from such esteemed publications as the *Journal of the American Medical Association, The New England Journal of Medicine, Archives of Internal Medicine,* and other professional organizations.

Scientific research has established that your beliefs, your expectations, and your emotional state can actually make as much of (if not more than) a difference as more physiological manipulations. In other words (to toss out a bumper-sticker simplification of our thesis), doctors don't always heal people; people often heal themselves.

If you can tap in to those positive health-promoting internal pathways and circumvent negative influences and expectations, you can go a long way toward healing and prevention without creating a need for frequent medical intervention. We are not recommending that you forsake competent professional medical care in hopes that you can somehow "trick" yourself into feeling better.

How This Book Is Organized
The writing of this book was prompted by the virtual explosion of information on factors that influence our immune system—and hence, our health. We provide an overview of the Immunity-

Pleasure Connection, including what it is and what brought the medical and scientific community to the doorstep of this exciting concept. We present a very basic description and explanation of the various parts of the immune system and how they function, followed by a look at the ways in which our mental disposition and stress put our systems at risk.

We also present laboratory, clinical, and field research, both recently published as well as some as-yet-unpublished findings, as they relate to pertinent health-related issues. These findings support the premise that you can influence your immune system by fine-tuning your body's major pleasure pathways. Much of the writing is drawn from approximately 18 years of research and addresses the influence of various psychosocial and environmental phenomena upon immune system function. We also introduce a revolutionary new proposition: that the immune system influences us psychologically.

We have steadfastly attempted to consider only scientific studies, not anecdotal evidence. As unusual as some of the studies we describe may sound, they were, indeed, real studies. If they had obvious weaknesses, we point them out. In some spots, we speculate beyond the data.

And, we show you how to get connected, literally, by integrating the Immunity-Pleasure Connection into your daily life. Throughout the book, we provide a variety of pleasure formulas that you can use to accomplish this. These are practical, easily accomplished real-world suggestions for how you can mobilize your body's own self-defense forces against illness by taking advantage of your natural affinity for sex, pets, music, laughter, and loved ones, among other matters. Plus, we offer a taste of how easy and delightful immune system enhancement is with a 13-Point Pleasure Formula.

Finally, an end-of-book glossary groups common immunity terms and their definitions in one place for easy reference.

So, are we saying that if you have sex, listen to some music, get a dog, and enjoy a few laughs, you'll never get sick? Of course not.

You could do every single thing we suggest throughout the book and still get a cold or still develop cancer. We are not saying that pleasurable behaviors are the only influences on the immune system. What we are saying is that pleasurable activities can give the immune system a meaningful and much-needed boost. Some of these boosts might be modest, but remember: Boosts can add up. Small increases in immune function, delivered simultaneously from several sources, together add up to a large boost. And this may be all it takes to tip the scales from "sick" to "not sick."

The British philosopher Thomas Hobbes was famous for saying that life was "nasty, brutish, and short." Aside from not sounding like a prime candidate to share a beer with, we think Hobbes was wrong. We believe that life can be wonderful, pleasurable, and long. The human drive for pleasure, if satisfied in moderation, can assist us on the pathway to good health. What a fantastic notion that is!

The Immunity-Pleasure Connection

WHAT IT IS, HOW IT WORKS—
AND HOW IT CAN WORK FOR YOU

Humanity has advanced, when it has advanced, not because it has been sober, responsible, and cautious, but because it has been playful, rebellious, and immature.
—Tom Robbins, novelist

As she has done for the past 2 weeks, Mary arrives at the office at the crack of dawn. Her husband is not at all happy about her unusually early workday hours of late. They have argued about it more than once, but she has no other choice. The fights they have had linger in her mind as she walks into the office cafeteria, makes a pot of coffee, gets a breakfast bar from the vending machine, reports to her desk, rubs her eyes to wake up, and begins to work.

An hour or so later, a colleague comes in. He leans over Mary's desk to discuss a document, yawns, and then sneezes. She instinctively pulls back; her colleague apologizes profusely but continues

1

to sniffle. They return their attention to the document. Mary realizes that she might have been exposed to some contaminated air, but she tells herself that the exposure was brief and inconsequential. After all, already well into the cold-and-flu season, she has managed to avoid falling ill. Besides, she is too overwhelmed with other matters to worry about getting sick.

What Mary fails to realize, though, is that she has been upping her odds of getting a cold all morning.

Let us retrace her steps: She touched likely germ-contaminated door handles and elevator buttons on her way to the office. She pressed another button on the vending machine, another probable source of contamination. Then she rubbed her eyes, allowing any germs or viruses present to gain entry via one of the most vulnerable parts of her body. Her hands also touched the breakfast bar before it entered her mouth, another vulnerable entry point. And then there was that sneeze.

If Mary were free from all other worries, she probably would remain invulnerable to the flu. But she is so fraught with an assortment of psychological concerns that she ultimately does succumb to the bug. Stress, intense concern with self, and disturbed family dynamics increase our chances of getting sick by compromising the immune system's ability to respond and protect, increasing the penetrability of our mucus membranes and strengthening the reproductive prowess of viruses and bacteria.

Mary may blame her sneezy coworker for making her ill, but odds are that as long as she fails to control the world around her—and fails to inject some much-needed TLC into her life—she is going to get sick again . . . and soon.

Making the Connection

Researchers are finding that what we call the mind—that mystical entity that includes thoughts, memories, emotions, and personality—is related to the activity of high-level brain neurons that make descending connections to other neurons lower in the brain, then in the spinal cord, and ultimately out in the rest of the body. This belief, held by most modern neuroscientists, has been explored in a book called *The Astonishing Hypothesis* by Nobel Prize–winner Sir Francis Crick. According to Crick and others, these "end neurons" can influence all aspects of the immune system, from B and T cells to lymph organs such as the spleen and thymus. This esoteric neuroanatomical fact has enormous ramifications for health care. Here, in a few connections, is a relatively simple pathway whereby things like mood, personality, and behavior can alter immune activity.

The notion that the mind can influence our health is really not new. Physicians as far back as 2nd-century Rome observed a relationship between depressed mood and later development of cancer. "The worry and strain of modern times contributes greatly to arterial degeneration," said the world-famous cardiologist Sir William Osler. It is an interesting mind-body statement, but all the more interesting because it was made in 1898! Such statements began to surface in the medical literature as early as the 18th century, and by Osler's time, scientific demonstrations of the mind-body connection started to appear.

From the middle 1900s on, medicine generally has chosen to focus most of its attention on the body, not the mind, emphasizing surgery and pharmacology at the expense of psychology. While many people—doctors and patients alike—believed that there was indeed a connection between state of mind and state of health, little supporting documented evidence ever existed or was pursued. Contributing to the lack of evidence was a basic scientific presumption that the immune system somehow operates separately from the body's other physiological systems.

Mind-body studies never went away, however. They were merely submerged under the general labels of "behavioral medicine" and "psychosomatic medicine." And in the past few decades, as science and technology have advanced, researchers have become able to establish absolutely that far from functioning independently of the rest of the body, the immune system interacts intimately and extensively with the nervous system, which governs all of our thoughts and physiological processes, and the endocrine system, which secretes hormones. Thoughts affect hormones, hormones affect thoughts, thoughts affect immune components, and hormones affect immune components in an impossibly complicated interrelationship the depth of which science is only just beginning to fathom. One statement that we can make with a high degree of certainty is that the existence of these direct pathways between mind and immunity is clear. And that's the thinking that gave birth to the Immunity-Pleasure Connection.

Psychoneuroimmunology: A Mouthful of Mind Medicine

This fundamental concept—that the immune system is an entity that we can proactively manage rather than reactively medicate—has led researchers to discover and document a number of ways that variables other than good old-fashioned germs can compromise our health. For example, it is now widely accepted that high stress and low moods weaken our defenses, making us more susceptible not only to the flu but also to such major problems as heart disease and cancer.

The volume of such newly acquired evidence is so extensive, in fact, that it has led to a whole new field of medicine devoted to immune system interactions with the mind and the progression of disease. It has been dubbed *psychoneuroimmunology*, a mouthful of a name that refers to psychology (*psycho*), the brain and nervous system (*neuro*), and your personal civil defense force, the immune system (*immunology*). To avoid stumbling over this tongue twister, we refer to psychoneuroimmunology as PNI.

Here is some of the research that substantiates this growing body of knowledge about behavioral medicine, of which PNI is an integral part.

◆ Consider the Houston orthopedic surgeon who took up the cases of 10 candidates for arthroscopic knee surgery. On 5 of the participants, he performed the actual procedure. On the other 5 willing subjects, he simply pretended to perform surgery by making three simple incisions. After 6 months, all 10 patients felt a substantial reduction in knee pain.

◆ In Seattle, a cardiologist operated on a group of people with the chest pains of angina pectoris. Ninety percent felt fewer chest pains upon exertion. For another group of people with angina, the cardiologist told them that he would operate, but he merely made superficial chest incisions and immediately sutured them up. Afterward, 90 percent of the people with the sham surgery—all of whom knew they were part of a study—said that they experienced fewer chest pains.

◆ A British physician studied the mind's and body's potential for self-healing among 200 people with nonspecific, nonserious conditions. To half of the people he offered diagnoses and told them that they would be better in a few days. To the others he said that he did not know why they felt ill and could not predict when their symptoms would clear. Two weeks later, 64 percent of those in the first group, who were reassured and comforted, had recovered from their maladies. In contrast, only 39 percent of the people left hanging for a prognosis had felt better.

◆ And then there's the study conducted by researcher F. J. Evans involving hospital patients who were in sufficiently great pain to warrant injections of morphine, the powerful opium-derived narcotic. All were told that they would receive the drug, but morphine was administered only to some of them. The others received a placebo containing no pain-relieving potential whatsoever. Those injected with the inert substance enjoyed 56 percent of the pain relief of those who received the actual morphine.

The point is, it was their minds and not some wonder drug that brought many of the test subjects the relief that they were seeking. In fact, much of modern pharmacy's effectiveness—anywhere from

35 percent to 75 percent, depending upon the drug in question, the research procedures followed, and whose statistics are used—has been scientifically attributed to nothing more than the simple belief that taking a pill will work. This phenomenon has come to be known as the placebo effect.

The Common Denominator: Pleasure

As described by Nathaniel S. Lehrman, M.D., in 1993 in the *Archives of Internal Medicine*, "The placebo effect is one of the most important examples of the principle that pleasure heals." This, of course, begs the question, How does it work?

Physiologically, psychologically, neurologically, and immunologically, placebo administration affects the body and mind much like stress reduction.

- ◆ It calms the health-damaging hormonal and chemical turbulence that stress induces.
- ◆ It triggers a counteractive health-improving flow of feel-good chemicals.
- ◆ The feel-good chemicals fortify the strength of the immune system.

According to a provocative, growing body of research, your immune system doesn't know (or care) what the source of the placebo is. Whether you were treated with a fake drug, a sham surgical procedure, or a healthy dose of cuddling, laughing, and Chardonnay is beside the point; in each case, the mind can triumph over matter.

The Natural High: In Tune with the Immune System

To understand what accounts for the placebo effect, it helps to take a look at some of the studies relating to the state that we know as happiness. What, physiologically, produces this unique state of mind? Considerable research has concentrated on the central nervous system's release of endorphins, enkephalins, dynorphins, and other similar substances. These chemicals, often collectively (and simplistically) referred to as endorphins, are classified as opioid peptides or endogenous (naturally produced) opiates. As the name implies, they look (in terms of chemical structure) and act (albeit to a much milder and safer extent) like opium, the poppy-derived narcotic that has been used and abused since 4000 B.C. or so to relax, sedate, kill pain, elicit pleasurable feelings, and induce euphoria.

For a little evidence, let us return to the study involving morphine, which is the stronger pharmaceutical version of the poppy-plant extract. Recall that pain abated by more than half for the people who were under the false impression that they had received an injection of the actual drug. When doctors administered chemicals (such as naloxone or naltrexone) that block the effects of both naturally secreted and externally administered opioids, no such relief occurred. Presumably, their faith in the bogus morphine treatment caused them to secrete their own endogenous opiates. (By the way, naloxone is commonly used as an antidote to narcotic overdoses, while naltrexone, under the brand name ReVia, has been used to help people overcome narcotic addiction.)

Endorphins are responsible for the so-called runner's high experienced with moderate exercise. And, as 18th century British physician John Jones pointed out in the *Journal of Neurology, Neurosurgery, and Psychiatry*, they are also associated with "a permanent gentle degree of that pleasure which modesty forbids the name of" (a.k.a. orgasm). Today, thanks to animal research, we now know that endorphin levels are some 86 times higher after animals experience multiple orgasms.

Our bodies do not secrete endorphins only as we work out or engage in sex. They also release them at times when we experience pleasure. It matters not whether we are playing with the family dog or cat, watching a funny movie, listening to our favorite music, rolling in the hay, rolling with the punches, seeing silver linings in

Blue, Red, or Green: What's Your Pleasure?

In Latin, the word *placebo* means "I will please." And given the extensive amount of research that pain researchers have done on the topic, it should come as no surprise that certain placebos please patients more than others. For example, white, angularly shaped pills are better at producing physiological effects than round white pills; colored tablets are more effective than white ones; and see-through capsules containing tiny hue-tinted beads are stronger inducers of an effect than colored tablets. A placebo is better received as a shot in the arm than as an orally administered agent, and an intravenous placebo treatment is more powerful than an injection. Finally, any placebo administered by a professional at a hospital is far more convincing than if you take it yourself at home.

dark clouds—or believing that some purported treatment is going to make us well again. All that the body knows is that, in some way, it is being satisfied.

We would be remiss if we ended our argument in favor of endogenous endorphins just with assertions that they counter immune-hampering stress hormones and improve mood. Pleasure chemicals do much more; they can actually improve immune function by producting an antibacterial peptide. They also enhance the killer instincts and abilities of various immune components, including B cells, T cells, NK cells, and immunoglobulins (all of which will be discussed in the next chapter). In fact, certain immune cells are able to secrete their own endorphins as a way of honing their lethal edge. In general, when your body releases endogenous opiates, your immune system is more active, more productive, more lethal, and more protective.

As scientists, we find all of these facts and their logical implications astoundingly significant. At least to some extent, certain inducements of happiness, joy, contentment, and pleasure can enhance traditional therapies.

Chapter 1

Say Hello to Your Immune System

YOUR BODY'S DEPARTMENT OF DEFENSE

Winning isn't everything. It's the only thing.
—Vince Lombardi, former Green Bay Packers coach

If you could put under a microscope all the food you eat, the water you drink, the air you breathe, and everything that your hands and body touch, you'd be so shocked, scared, repulsed, and disgusted that you'd want to live in a disinfected, impenetrable bubble. The sheer number of bugs, germs, microorganisms, and other nasty substances looking to set up house inside your body is astounding. They're everywhere. Their efforts are unrelenting, and you can't escape them.

Bacteria, viruses, cancer-encouraging chemicals, fungi, parasites—they all want you, or at least a piece of you. Many are harmless, but others can drain the life right out of you. (All of them are known collectively as antigens. Those that can make us ill are called pathogens. See "Know Your Enemy" on page 22.) To protect your body, nature developed a surefire strategy: Develop an internal defense system in which anything that doesn't naturally belong in the body will be identified, attacked, and hopefully destroyed.

Welcome to your immune system, a 24-hour-a-day operation designed solely to keep you healthy and alive. How well it works is another matter entirely. It's composed of obscure substances, intricate interrelationships, contradictions, and other technicalities. The immune system certainly is complicated, but a basic understanding of how it functions is fundamental to grasping why the pleasurable things in life preserve your health.

The War on Bugs: How the Immune System Operates

The immune system is a complex network of cells and organs. The B-cell system, consisting largely of a handful of constantly circulating antibodies called immunoglobulins, comprises your humoral immunity. The various T cells are part of what's known as cellular immunity. The organs that generate these fluids and cells include bone marrow; the thymus, which is located in the front of your chest cavity; the lymph nodes, found in your neck, under your arms, and elsewhere in your upper trunk; and a coalition called mucosal-associated lymphoid tissue (MALT), which consists of your tonsils, adenoids, appendix, and Peyer's patches in the intestines.

How does it all work? Consider this military metaphor: Aerial reconnaissance detects an enemy advance on a strategically valuable piece of land and radios an alert to headquarters. Headquarters signals a crack platoon of roving sentries on the perimeter of the territory to be ready for battle. Despite their often-accurate aim in picking off and halting intruders, a particularly crafty and diligent enemy cadre manages to penetrate this initial defensive line. The sentries signal gung-ho guards from other stationed squads for further assistance. These infantrymen do what they can

Immune System Organs

We all know that our bodies have organs and tissue that provide us with the immune protection we need. But who can name them all, much less pinpoint their location? Here's a quick primer to help you get to know your immune system better.

Primary

Bone marrow: inner area of all bones
Thymus: front of chest cavity

Secondary

Lymph nodes: between neck and pelvis
Spleen: trunk area

Mucosal-Associated Lymphoid Tissue

Tonsils: oral cavity
Adenoids: oral cavity
Appendix: trunk area
Peyer's patches: intestines

to beat back the attack but are forced to call for more help. Soon, other ruthless warriors, some with bayonets, charge in and stab or otherwise kill the trespassers. At the same time, other units, sensing trouble, may have already joined the fray in helping to win one for our side.

The battlefield metaphor may be a cliché in describing how the immune system functions, but it's accurate on several levels. Whether on the front line or inside the body, the goal remains the same: Kill and eliminate the enemy. The stakes are the same, too: Lose the war, and the consequences could very well be deadly. Each of the military players in the muddy, bloody battlefield analogy above has an immune system counterpart with similar duties.

Inspecting the Troops

Each part of the immune system has its own separate functions, but all interact with one another via chemical and neural signals in an intricate chain of command and communication that involves cells, enzymes, hormones, and brain chemicals.

Humoral immunity. The fluid-based humoral immune system, utilizing the bloodstream and all mucosal tissue secretions, is comprised of antibodies, the most prevalent of which is immunoglobulin A (IgA). It represents your body's initial defensive counterattack when an antigen attempts to invade. It's the perimeter-patrolling sentinel that's always on alert and ready to halt any intruder immediately upon detection. Except for a tiny two-tenths of one percent of us, everyone is born with IgA and so-called innate immunity. (Another kind of internal defense, called acquired immunity, develops depending on our individual unique exposures to various antigens.)

Cellular immunity. These various warriors, white blood cells housed mostly in bone marrow and the thymus, both communicate and eradicate. They include the radio reconnaissance flyers, the commanders at headquarters who notify the humoral sentinels, and the killers that help deliver the final blow against the enemy.

The reticuloendothelial system (RES). If the roaming antibody sentinels don't immediately stop the invasion, these specialized sentinels, stationed at specific strategic points deeper within the defensive perimeter, take aim and fire. RES is comprised of all the lymphocytes produced by the lymph nodes, the spleen, and MALT, plus certain white blood cells (monocytes and macrophages) manufactured in bone marrow. These guards will try to stop anything that gets past the initial sentries along the outer perimeter.

Nonspecific effector system. More backup killers deeper in the territory, these white blood cells, organized into units called monocytes, macrophages, neutrophils, and natural killer cells, also charge out of bone marrow and into the bloodstream. They act on intuition, attacking whenever they sense danger.

Complement. These ruthless proteins and enzymes, called up from the humoral barracks, are specialized killers armed with the cellular equivalent of bayonets. They charge in and quite literally poke a hole in the infectious invader's cell membrane, killing it.

Humoral Immunity: No Laughing Matter

Except for when you suffer a laceration, the only real way for a microorganism to invade the body and threaten your health is through soft, penetrable, moist, mucosal areas—the eyes, nose, mouth, genital openings, and rectum. It first must pass through the very outermost layer of mucus (the mucosal lumen), then attempt to penetrate the mucosal epithelium before entering tissue cells and the bloodstream. This puts the fluid-based humoral immune system on the front line and immunoglobulins in leading roles as the body's initial defenders.

The onus falls heavily on IgA. It's the star player here. Though also found in the bloodstream, IgA is most heavily concentrated in the fluids of our most vulnerable places: tears, mucus, saliva, and vaginal and prostatic secretions. It also appears in breast milk. Get comfortable with this crucially important immune substance. We'll turn our attention to it frequently throughout the book. It not only combats illness but it also deters illness from starting in the first place. When a foreign substance is first detected, IgA rushes in, binds to it, and prevents it from further entering the body. If the antigen somehow evades this first defensive line, IgA signals other immune system phagocytes to step in and literally devour the intruder. A phagocyte is any cell that engulfs and enzymatically degrades an intruder. (The term *phagocyte* comes from the Greek word *phagein*, meaning "to eat." Phagocytosis is the process by which cells from other immune subsystems consume foreign cells.)

A quartet of other immunoglobulins also exists. They're present in far smaller concentrations (we have more IgA than the other four combined) and possess limited, specific duties. Immunoglobulin M (IgM), for instance, works in the bloodstream and is the first immunoglobulin that appears after antigen exposure. It binds to any invading antigens and signals for help from other immune components. Its appearance is quite brief, though, and it soon cedes responsibility for longer-term protection to immunoglobulin G (IgG). The primary duty of immunoglobulin E (IgE) is to trigger the production of histamine (and the resulting sniffling, sneezing, wheezing, and tearing) during an allergic reaction. It also participates in the destruction of parasites. The functions of immunoglobulin D (IgD), unfortunately, are largely unknown.

Cellular Immunity: When the Going Gets Tough

From where do IgA and the other immunoglobulins come? How are they deployed for infection-protection jobs? For answers, we need to step out of the saliva and mucus and jump into the bones and bloodstream.

The two major components of the cellular immune system, B lymphocytes and T lymphocytes (for the sake of simplicity, we'll call them B cells and T cells), are white blood cells manufactured in bone marrow. B cells stay there to mature before being deployed, while T cells migrate to the thymus to grow. Generally, both types of lymphocytes play roles in detecting invaders, maintaining a sort of institutional memory of all intruders ever encountered and developing the immune system's ability to both specialize and diversify in eradicating any imaginable outsider.

B Cells: Transforming, Remembering

B lymphocytes work mostly outside the body's other cells and identify bacteria. When an unknown intruder breaks down the door, helper T cells ring the bell and wake up B cells. Once the alarm goes off, B cells release themselves rapidly into the bloodstream and

Play Cards

Contract bridge apparently can increase your number of T lymphocytes. A presentation at the annual meeting of the Society for Neuroscience in 2000 by Marian Cleeves Diamond of the University of California, Berkeley, involved data from blood samples taken before and after 90 minutes of bridge playing. The participants were 12 women, all in their 70s and 80s, 4 of whom showed slight increases in their amounts of T lymphocytes—cells in the immune system that discriminate between the body's own cells and anything that might be alien—while 8 showed significant increases in T cell counts.

The speculation is that the game involves planning functions, working memory, sorting and sequencing tasks, and initiative. These are all functions of the dorsolateral portion of the frontal lobe of the brain's cortex, and some research suggests that this part of the brain is involved in immune system function. If this is the case, the likelihood is that any game that produces this sort of mental activity will produce similar results. This may be a small piece of the correlation that we find in other studies between intelligence and good health. Or it could be the mere pleasure that one derives from the game that does the trick, or perhaps a combination of these variables.

signal IgA, IgD, IgE, IgG, and IgM antibodies throughout our mucosal linings and the blood. The immunoglobulins then bind themselves to the intruder and, if necessary, emit an SOS to other immune system troops.

Like elephants, B cells never forget. They carry most of the immune system's institutional memory of previous engagements. When an antigen is encountered and a specific antibody is created to destroy it, B cells house the information and instinctively know what to do every other time that specific intruder dares to cross the threshold. As opposed to the general, all-purpose innate immunity with which each of us enters the world, this specialization is known as acquired immunity. All of us acquire our own unique immune arsenals depending on our different encounters with the enemy world. The concept of inoculating us against diseases is based on deliberately introducing a harmless, "innocuous" amount of a pathogen precisely so that B cells can react, learn, and remember how to produce antibodies effective enough to fight it. Thank B cells and acquired immunity for the success of Jonas Salk's polio shot and all of our other vaccines.

T Cells: Helping, Killing

Working primarily inside our other cells, T cells are charged with discriminating between the body's own cells and anything that might be alien. They also identify the presence of a virus and note any changes in the shape of our cells that might signal the development of cancer. Two basic types of these lymphocytes develop during the maturation stage in the thymus gland: cytotoxic T cells, which are out-and-out killers that engage in phagocytosis, and helper T cells, which carry the phagocytes to infection sites and provoke inflammation (hence the swelling that we get around a cut). These T cells also are responsible for alerting B cells to step into the intruder-stopping fray.

During the maturation process, both B cells and T cells are twice inspected by other cells to guarantee that they function correctly and can properly distinguish between the body's own cells and any other foreign matter. For T cells, this inspection stage is especially crucial. Any slipup that allows abnormal T cells into the ranks spells big trouble—namely, an autoimmune disorder. T cells that don't know the difference between an invader and your body's own naturally occurring cells are going to wreak havoc on your health.

Those T cells that pass initial inspection become part of our genes by binding to a segment of DNA called the major histocompatability complex (MHC). With more than 100 subclasses and permutations, they then become either permanent parts of our every cell or immune system specialists. The two most important things to keep in mind are CD4 T cells and CD8 T cells. CD4 cells are helper T cells that promote inflammation; CD8 cells are cytotoxic T cells that kill and sometimes rein in and suppress immune system activity.

The RES-t of the Story

Out of both the lymphatic system and bone marrow come the monocytes and macrophages that comprise RES. Wherever an infection arises, monocytes are generated in large numbers, and they transform themselves into macrophages that circulate throughout the body looking for something to destroy. The name of these roving sentries means "big eaters." They literally engulf and consume antigens. Other specialized white blood cells that live to eat belong to the nonspecific effector system, which, besides monocytes and macrophages, includes monocytes, neutrophils, and natural killer cells (NK cells). They remain on continuous, nonstop search-and-destroy missions throughout the body. Rounding out your internal armed forces are the serum proteins of complement. These fierce, merciless assassins latch on to antigens and release enzymes that poke fatal holes in the intruders' cell membranes. Complement proteins also present antigens to phagocytes, often when IgA is involved.

Cytokines: How the Mind Practices Medicine

The choreography required to present this dance against disease is mind-boggling. Proteins, enzymes, hormones, brain neurotransmitters, and other cells communicate with one another through an elaborate chemical and neural network. The fact of the matter is that the chemical changes that occur when we are sick often are the same chemical movements that occur when we are stressed, depressed, or otherwise emotionally low. This is the basis for our proposition that mood, disposition, mental state, and degree of pleasure in one's life exert a profound impact on our ability to remain free of illness.

The great facilitators here, the main molecules that activate, tone down, and otherwise regulate immune activity, are called cytokines. These polypeptide hormones, as they're called, come in a number of varieties: interferon, transformational growth factor (TGF), some 18 different interleukins, and several types of tumor necrosis factor (TNF). Whenever a pathogen or other stressor strikes, cytokines appear on the scene to jump-start the immune system, promote inflammation, and initiate the "acute phase response" of sickness. The so-called pro-inflammatory cytokines (including interleukin-1, interleukin-6, and TNF) are particularly important because of their prominent presence in illness and other disorders. Interleukin-1, for example, helps generate a fever and involves itself in the release of prostaglandin E2, which contributes to controlling pain. It also regulates activity in the hypothalamic part of the brain that governs a whole host of biological and psychological functions.

Interleukin-6, another pro-inflammatory cytokine, plays key roles in telling B cells to get to work generating antibodies, and in helping to make interleukin-1 much more potent in carrying out its various duties. It also shows up when we are ill, when we are under a lot of stress, and when we are depressed. Another factor is interleukin-2, which, along with interleukin-1 and interleukin-6, shows up not only among people with an infection but among people with schizophrenia (see "The 'New' Infectious Diseases" on page 25). TNF contributes to generating a fever, and it enhances the secretion of stress-associated catecholamines. Interestingly enough, TNF's presence also is associated with memory and attention.

Flu or Blue?

Whether you are depressed, severely stressed, or just really sick, the effects on and reactions by your body are basically the same. Below are the various symptoms that your body displays when you are injured or struck down with the flu. Many of these same symptoms also occur when you are depressed or experiencing a considerable amount of tension.

◆ Fever

◆ Increased slow-wave (non-rapid eye movement) sleep

◆ Alterations in plasma iron

◆ Shifts in protein synthesis

◆ Increased levels of white blood cells

◆ Diminished thirst

◆ Diminished appetite

◆ Increased sensitivity to pain

◆ Reduced activity

◆ Reduced exploration (curiosity-induced activity)

◆ Decreased aggression

◆ Decreased sexual desire

◆ Diminished interest and pleasure in activity

◆ Depressed mood

◆ Loss of attention

◆ Memory problems

◆ Release of stress hormones

Disease and Disposition

Note the correlation between the presence of cytokines and emotional state. Cytokines show up not only when we are physically sick but also when we are not well psychologically. This simple fact lays the foundation for the Immunity-Pleasure Connection and much of mind-body medicine.

Because of pro-inflammatory cytokines, the symptoms of having a bad cold and being depressed are similar (see "Flu or Blue?"). What this means is that in the presence of either a pathogen or severe emotional stress, the body reacts in virtually the same way. It means not only that stress can make you ill but also that, via cytokines and pathogens, your immune system can stress you out and affect you psychologically.

Understand that cytokines, in and of themselves, are not bad. On the contrary, they trigger immune activity and coordinate the show when we are physically sick. They become problematic, however, when secreted in overabundance, typically because of an immune system glitch instigated by emotional stress and strain.

For the moment, consider how stress facilitates a pathogen's ability to defeat our immune defenses. For instance, stress hormones change both the number and distribution of various immune cells, reducing resistance to an infection; drugs that suppress stress hormones can strengthen immune resistance. Stress alters the permeability of mucosal linings, giving pathogens easier entry into the body, the bloodstream, and the brain.

It's one thing to say that you can think yourself sick and make other assumptions about psychological influences on health. It's quite another thing to be able to document, thanks to the advent of psychoneuroimmunology, the physiological basis for such claims. Why would stress and a pathogen force the body to react in almost identical ways? What's the common denominator? In brief, from the immune system's perspective, the common denominator is a threat to good health and survival. From the earliest stages of mankind, the greatest threat to survival has come from microorganisms. That's how the immune system came into being, and the stress response may have evolved from that physical survival mechanism. Faced with any harrowing life-or-death situation, it's no wonder that the immune system would become involved.

The Internal Failure

With a basic understanding under our belts of how the immune system functions, let's turn to its failure to keep us healthy. Illness and disease occur for two reasons: The immune system is either too weak or otherwise impaired, or the strength or sheer numbers of certain pathogens simply overpowers it. The weakness and impairment could stem from either physical or psychological factors or a combination of both. The overwhelming opposition also could emerge from a combination of physical and psychological liabilities.

A discussion of diseases with which the immune system must cope could go on endlessly. Here are a few categories particularly susceptible to such factors as stress and the presence (or absence) of pleasure.

Autoimmune Diseases: The Enemy Within

"We have met the enemy and he is us," the immortal Walt Kelly wrote in his often scathing political parody comic strip *Pogo*. That pretty much sums up what's going on inside the bodies of people with an autoimmune disease, such as rheumatoid arthritis, lupus, multiple sclerosis, psoriasis, and ulcerative colitis.

If you have an autoimmune disease, you have an immune system that has gone awry and sees certain cells in your own body as foreign invaders that must be eradicated. Almost any organ or system in the body can be affected by this friendly fire. In multiple sclerosis, for example, the immune system thinks that the protective covering over your nerves is a foreign invader. In rheumatoid arthritis, it thinks that your joint cartilage is the bad guy. Addison's disease, Grave's disease, myasthenia gravis, pernicious anemia, rheumatic fever, scleroderma, type 1 diabetes—all are autoimmune disorders.

No one knows precisely or entirely why autoimmune disorders exist, why the presence of naturally occurring cells triggers the immune system to attack, or why the immune system can't distinguish between desired, needed, necessary body cells and unwanted, deleterious invader cells. Something goes horribly wrong in the body's "self code," a unique group of antigens called human leukocyte

Know Your Enemy

From what does the immune system protect us? Cell-destroying, cancer-causing substances represent one category to which our internal guard devotes a considerable portion of its resources. Aside from a few stray invaders that aren't easily classified, the other main illness-causing pathogens are bacteria, viruses, fungi, and parasites, with bacteria and viruses the predominant threats.

Bacteria. These one-celled organisms are the tiniest creatures capable of eating, developing, and reproducing by themselves. The immune system typically is very capable of seeking out and destroying bacteria. In some cases, however (pneumonia and the bubonic plague, to name two good examples), the sheer number encountered and the speed of reproduction leave the immune system with its hands full. While this was a deadly problem in the past, the advent of sulfa drugs and antibiotics just before the mid 1900s has, for the most part, eliminated the possibility of death from these organisms. You can still get sick, but you probably won't die.

Viruses. These differ greatly from bacteria. They consist of complex molecules found in all cells of the body, either DNA or RNA, and have no life of their own. They're able to survive and multiply only by infecting and taking over host cells. Medications and vaccines have been created to help fight off some viruses, especially some of the more debilitating ones, but the immune system by and large does a good job of protecting us from these bugs.

Fungi. Molds, yeasts, and other life forms in this category usually don't cause major immune or other health-related problems. True, yeast infections can be nagging and uncomfortable, but only rarely are they very serious.

Parasites. These organisms must rely on another living thing for survival, usually to the detriment of the host. Nowadays, we usually acquire parasitic infections from poorly prepared food.

group A (HLA) that's present in almost every cell and determined by the major histocompatability complex (MHC), whose job it is to transport all things that shouldn't be there (nonself) to the cellular surface for detection and eradication by our immune armies. In an autoimmune disorder, immune cells, primarily T cells, in the MHC fail to distinguish between external invading cells and instead bind to natural self cells, setting off an immune response that clobbers the self cells. The glitch can arise in several ways.

◆ Various "tricky" bacteria and viruses are able to pass themselves off as certain self cells, avoid immediate detection, and set up shop in the body. The masquerade won't last long, though; the immune system will ultimately realize the deception. However, in its zeal to eradicate the invaders and not be fooled again, it aggressively and indiscriminately attacks the tricky antigens and anything else that looks similar, including self cells.

◆ Chemicals or radiation exposure can initiate autoimmune disorders by altering self cells and making them appear unnatural, or by altering immune cells so that they begin to manufacture antibodies to self cells.

◆ In other instances, certain injuries trigger the destructive reaction. For reasons not wholly understood, a few parts of the body, primarily the eyes, the testes, and the heart, are not directly protected by IgA, B cells, T cells, and the rest of our defense forces. Immune cells swim all around these organs, but none exist inside them. So when there's a direct physical injury to one of these spots, immune cells immediately rush in, but they cannot distinguish between what cells are alien and what cells should naturally exist. Mired in the uncertainty, they start killing indiscriminately. In other words, if you poke your eye with a pencil, get stabbed in the heart, or somehow rupture a testicle, your immune system might cause big trouble.

◆ Nature wasn't entirely stupid; it did provide for suppressor T cells to help control the destruction if something goes awry with immune function. While this fail-safe mechanism usually works, it too can become defective.

AIDS: Outsmarting Immunity

The trickiest, most cunning virus known is the human immunodeficiency virus (HIV) that causes acquired immunodeficiency syndrome (AIDS). Instead of attacking an organ or a nerve or another body part, it specifically targets the immune system, primarily our helper and inflammatory CD4 T cells. The virus gets a foothold in a horribly deceptive yet bafflingly simple ruse that, amazingly enough, fools the immune system. Once inside a CD4 T cell, one of its ploys is to rotate and turn itself sideways, so to speak. That little dodge is enough to make itself invisible to our vast internal armed forces, enough to dupe the immune system into thinking the cell is uncontaminated. Undetected, the virus replicates itself and spreads in wildly mutational ways throughout the immune system. Medications and immune components able to counteract one eventually detected strain of the virus quickly are unable to oppose its next mutated form. At the same time, because the victim is the immune system itself, the body's defense mechanism falters, giving bacteria, unrelated viruses, and other opportunistic infections a newfound deadly potential.

By creating antibodies and cytotoxic T cells to kill infected cells, a healthy immune system that's functioning on peak power can, in fact, mount a defense against HIV for years. Read on to find out what you can do to elevate your overall emotional state to give yourself a better chance to resist the disease as researchers race for a cure.

Cancer: When Natural Becomes Unnatural

When abnormal cells arise in the body and disfigure other cells as they replicate and spread, the result is cancer. Half of all men and one-third of all women, according to estimates, are likely to develop some form of cancer at some point in their lives. It can hit virtually any part of the body, assume myriad forms, and progress in a multiplicity of ways. Mistakes in normal replication can mutate a cell and initiate a malignancy. So can exposure to radiation, viruses, and a variety of chemicals. Sometimes the immune system can battle the virulent spread; sometimes it's overwhelmed by the abnormal cells' speed and ruthless determination. Stress and certain emotional characteristics can exert a profound influence on the immune system's ability to combat the disease.

The "New" Infectious Diseases

Ulcers, heart attacks, depression, autism, and schizophrenia are hardly new health problems. What's new is the accumulating evidence that they may arise in the presence of certain pathogens or an immune system weakness.

We should tread cautiously here. If, for example, a black cat crosses your path and you soon get hit by a truck, it doesn't necessarily mean that the cat's appearance caused your misfortune. It doesn't mean that you can predict future disaster. It may simply be a coincidence. More abstractly, even if X and Y frequently occur together, you cannot conclude that one causes the other. X might cause Y; Y might cause X. However, Z or some other unknown factor may cause both. The most we can assert is that the presence of X predicts, to some degree, the presence of Y and vice versa. Scientists call this relationship a positive correlation.

So is a heart attack the result of an infection? Researchers in the United States and Finland have discovered disproportionate amounts of an odd bacteria-virus hybrid, called *Chlamydia pneumoniae*, in the arteries surrounding the hearts of people who have had coronaries. Other researchers have found no such large concentration, so the scientific jury is still out. If the infectious connection eventually comes to be true, the possibility remains that a healthy, happy, low-stress immune system may be better equipped to fend off this viral bacteria, thereby preventing a heart attack.

What about ulcers? Here, science is much more certain, knowing that the presence of *Helicobacter pylori* bacteria can account for holes in the gastrointestinal tract. But it's not as simple as that. About two-thirds of us harbor the bacteria; yet curiously, two-thirds of us do not have and will not get ulcers. What leaves people susceptible to the bug's erosive ways? The suspect is the same thing that always has been thought to cause an ulcer: stress. The thinking is that stress weakens the immune system in a way that allows *H. pylori* to inflict harm.

Autism as an immune dysfunction? Well, medicine once thought that the condition was entirely psychologically produced, but that hypothesis has been thoroughly discounted. Genetics has been thought to play some role, but it could not be the sole cause because this behavioral and psychosocial disorder has reached almost epidemic proportions in the United States, skyrocketing in incidence over the past decade from about 1 in 10,000 to 1 in 150, according to estimates released in 2000 by at least one study.

Other hypotheses have focused on the body's inability to process certain nutritional substances, and on exposure to certain environmental substances, and some evidence both directly and indirectly implicates the immune system. Some researchers have measured significant reductions of IgA and the complement's serum proteins and enzymes in people with autism. Other scientists have detected the presence of microorganisms in the brain that cause neural damage because of as-yet-unknown immune failures. Other work involves a combination of immune system activity and forms of depression and the brain chemical imbalances that they cause.

As for schizophrenia, evidence suggests that the thought aberrations stem from the body's inability to regulate the brain chemical dopamine properly. The presence of immune system cytokines (interleukin-1, interleukin-2, and interleukin-6) directly influences dopamine levels. People with schizophrenia often have elevated concentrations of these substances, and the higher presence has been

A Test of Competence

How is immune vitality calculated? Laboratories can easily perform a variety of tests. Some are quantitative, measuring numbers, amounts, or percentages of certain substances or cells; others are functional, judging ability to perform a given immune-related task.

In quantitative assessments, more is generally better. The more immunoglobulin A (IgA) in a saliva sample, for example, the better your immune system is working. The same is true for higher counts of B lymphocytes, T lymphocytes, natural killer cells, or neutrophils in a blood sample. Of the functional tests, one, another blood measure, involves incubating natural killer cells with tumor cells and noting the extent to which the cancerous cells are destroyed. The more that are murdered, of course, the stronger this aspect of immunity. Or lymphocytes, usually T cells, could be exposed to mitogens such as pokeweed mitogen, concanavalin A, or phytohemaglutinin. The better that the lymphocytes divide and replicate (*proliferate* is the technical term), the more effective the cellular immunity.

A few other tests don't rely on blood or saliva samples. In the so-called delayed-type hypersensitivity test, an antigen is injected under your skin, and the resulting inflammation is measured for an immune reaction. Here, the more inflammation observed, the better your immune health, because what's being gauged is how many inflammatory T cells arrive at the site to produce a cellular immune response. Similarly, you could be inoculated with an antigen and have antibody production measured. Again, in this judge of humoral immunity, the more antibodies, the better.

An indirect way to get an idea of immune system function is to assess antibody production to a latent virus. The herpesvirus is a good example. Once we are exposed to it—and it is a common, not necessarily sexually transmitted virus that almost all of us have been exposed to—it stays in the body forever, flaring up now and then when the immune system is suppressed, often (which should be of no surprise) during stressful times. When the virus becomes active and replicates, the body produces herpesvirus antibodies. The more antibodies present, the more the virus is becoming restless and about to wreak havoc.

associated with worsened symptoms of the disorder and a poorer prognosis. In fact, one study demonstrated that administering high doses of interleukin-2 produces several symptoms of the condition in otherwise emotionally healthy people.

There also may be a connection between immunity and obesity. In the summer of 2000, for example, scientists at the University of Wisconsin in Madison published a study showing that adenovirus-36 (a common human virus that typically causes colds, diarrhea, or pinkeye) makes chickens and mice obese. The infected animals didn't weigh all that much more, but their bodies ended up containing more than twice as much fat as their uninfected counterparts. Up to 30 percent of all overweight people, according to related research, harbor the virus, compared with just 5 percent of thinner people.

It has been suggested by some that obesity itself causes the health problems linked to being overweight. But could the actual culprit be a virus? Is the culprit the stress-related physiological changes that encourage the body to put on pounds? Is it the immune-suppressing stress generated by the desire to be thinner? No one knows, but the evidence is strong enough to surmise that obesity is a combination of several of these factors.

We've touched here upon just a handful of afflictions that potentially could be labeled infectious diseases. For example, preliminary research suggests a possible immune system ability to eliminate the accumulation of neural plaque in the brains of people with Alzheimer's disease. The pattern is that science continually discovers evidence of immune system involvement in more ways than ever thought possible, and in the most unlikely places. Given its increasing prominence in our health, we need to emphasize whatever activities will help assure its maximum performance.

Getting Connected . . .
with Enhanced Immunity

This entire book rests on the foundation that enjoying yourself and reducing stress will shore up your immune system's ability to deflect and defeat illness. Every second of your life involves a fight between good health and antigens intent on overcoming you. The stronger your immune system, the better equipped for battle you'll be. Aside from pleasure, what else might you do to pump up your immune system and keep the troops in tip-top shape? Several ideas come to mind.

Demand a psyche-savvy doctor. Your immune system obviously is involved in almost everything you might see a doctor about. What's less apparent, though, is that your immune system is significantly influenced by your doctor, even before he prescribes a medication or performs any therapeutic procedure. Physicians can contribute to or help alleviate stress, and they can support and bolster your sense of self. You want a doctor with a wonderful bedside manner and a keen understanding of the complexities, both physical and psychological, involved in maintaining and restoring your health.

Watch (and wash) those hands. Illness-encouraging microorganisms are everywhere. Wash your hands frequently with lots of sudsy warm water. Use antibacterial soap only occasionally, though, so those bugs do not develop their own immunity to it. And keep your hands and fingers, even if they're spotlessly clean, away from your mouth, eyes, and nose, three favorite mucosal entry points for antigens.

Feast your eyes on food. Science knows that nutrition and diet can have an enormous impact on immune health. Besides the biochemistry, there's the pleasure factor: Few things are more delightful to the senses—from the smell and taste to the mere mouthwatering look of the dish—than the occasional lavish, delicious meal.

Visit the land of Nod. Sleep helps you restore and refresh immunity. When possible, indulge in 7 to 8 hours of restful slumber.

Chapter 2

It's All in Your Head

HOW ATTITUDE, DISPOSITION, AND MOOD AFFECT YOUR IMMUNITY

I don't get angry, I just grow a tumor.
—Woody Allen, screenwriter, actor, and director

You haven't felt like eating for a while now. In fact, you've lost a little weight. You aren't going out and getting together with friends. You don't even want to see family. You haven't bothered to shower or comb your hair for the past several days. You don't feel like doing anything, whether fun or not. Why? Well, you're tired. You're not sleeping well. And you were up all night. All in all, you feel positively lousy.

What's the diagnosis? If you went to your doctor and listed these symptoms, he would probably say that you have a cold or maybe the flu. If you went to a psychologist, he would probably say that you're depressed.

If you came to us, we'd say that it could be either or both. If you asked your body, it likely would tell you that it doesn't matter because, just as with stress (more about that culprit in the next chapter), the bottom line is the same: Whether you have a bug or the blues, the reactions of your immune system are uncannily similar.

You can travel on this street in either direction. Sure, you could be down in the dumps (or angry or negative or feeling helpless) because you are ill, but you also could be ill because you are down in the dumps (or angry or negative or feeling helpless).

Mood Medicine

Disposition, attitude, emotional state, and certain personality traits exert enormous influence on immune health and thus on the progression of disease. Whether you are optimistic or pessimistic, how well you handle anger and negativity, how downhearted and dispirited you are, how much control you think you have over your life, and other characteristics of your emotional makeup—all of these predict your tendency to get sick and to what degree.

◆ Optimists live longer than pessimists.
◆ Depressed people have higher rates of disease than their less-dejected peers.
◆ People with rheumatoid arthritis who received psychological treatment showed less local inflammation.
◆ The less you are able to appreciate and revel in pleasurable activities, the more likely you are going to be depressed and, thus, have health problems.

You don't even have to be a certified cynic or a dictionary definition of a depressed person. Day-to-day, hour-to-hour fluctuations in mood also exert influence on your immune strength and on the odds that you'll get sick. You might be a generally carefree, cheery, and well-adjusted person, but if you happen to be angry, upset, or otherwise negative just minutes before you ran your hand along a stairway railing that harbors a flu virus, you are more likely to get a cold than if you were happy-go-lucky and hostility-free when you came into contact with the bug. You will also remain sicker longer and feel sicker than you otherwise would have if you had been in a better frame of mind.

Once in a Blue Mood?

The notion that low spirits and unhealthy emotions influence disease has been more widely entertained than you might guess, and it's not at all new. Way back in the 2nd century, the ancient, eminent Roman physician Galen noted that "melancholic" women were more likely to develop breast cancer.

By the 1700s, the medical literature was replete with similar statements regarding mood and health, particularly in connection with cancer. For instance, noted surgeon Richard Guy, M.D., wrote in 1759 that women with cancer tend to be "of a sedentary, melancholic disposition of mind." Another 18th-century physician, Gendton, described the case of a woman who lived a life of perfect health until her daughter died. Afterward, she "underwent great affliction" and eventually noticed a swelling in her breast that "broke out in a most inveterate cancer."

The observations continued into the 1800s. In 1870, James Paget, M.D., described the so-called cancerous constitution, a condition in which "deep anxiety, deferred hope, and disappointment are frequently followed by the growth and increase of cancer." Another 19th-century physician, Walshe, wrote about the "influence of mental misery, sudden reversals of fortune, and habitual gloomings of the temper on the disposition of carcinomatous matter."

By the early 1890s, more scientifically oriented information began to supplant the anecdotal observations. Herbert Snow, M.D., of the London Cancer Hospital, conducted the very first statistically based study on cancer and psychological makeup. After analyzing data on 250 women with both breast and uterine cancers, he concluded, "the number of instances in which malignant disease of the breast and uterus follows immediate antecedent emotion of a depressing character is too large to be set down to chance."

Throughout the early and middle parts of the 20th century, similar references were made to the relationships between mood and disease. But from the mid 1900s on, medicine acquired more and more knowledge of the physiological and, as a consequence, placed increasingly less emphasis on the mind. The more that experts learned about how the body functions, the less they addressed how the mind might sway the body. Now medicine is stepping back for a look at the bigger picture through the prism of psychoneuroimmunology.

Optimism vs. Pessimism: Half Full or Half Empty?

You know Bob, or someone like him. He's the most steadfastly optimistic person you've ever met. Bob may be bankrupt, alone, and devoid of any prospects for improvement. His hair could be on fire, too, yet he views the blaze as the perfect opportunity to go out for a walk in the rain. Nothing ever seems to get this guy down. He is convinced that everything will turn around any time now. He never seems to get sick, either.

You also know Ellen: nice, sweet, generous—and the most pessimistic doomsayer you've ever encountered. She's the anti-Bob. Even when life is great, Ellen is convinced that misery lurks around the corner. She's certain that good things are nature's way of getting her to let her guard down so that disaster can strike. She's so negative that her doctor scribbled out a prescription for Prozac (fluoxetine hydrochloride). Ellen also seems to have some sort of health-related concern every day. Two days ago it was the ache in her belly. Yesterday it was a headache. You can safely bet that she's still not going to feel well tomorrow, either.

Ellen's glass of immunity-boosting immunoglobulin A (IgA) is half empty and draining fast; Bob's glass of IgA is at least half full, perhaps brimming.

Why? Because your disposition and overall outlook on life influence your immune system and your health in ways that the average doctor never would imagine. If you are pessimistic about your lot in life, science suggests, you can create a self-fulfilling prophecy that leads to disease.

We're back on the two-way street again. Yes, if you are successful, good-looking, healthy, and happy, you are probably going to be generally optimistic about life. But those assets aren't prerequisites for an upbeat outlook. No matter how dire your lot, just being optimistic engenders success, health, and happiness. In other words, being an optimist or a pessimist doesn't merely reflect how healthy or successful you are currently; it actually predicts your future health and your success in all aspects of life—how well you do in school, how much money you make, how stable your relationships will be. The more science investigates, the more confidently we can say that disposition determines health.

Scaling (or Plummeting from) Mount Optimism

Is your glass half-empty or half-full? Do you see the silver lining or only storm clouds? Here's a quick way to test your tendency.

Recall the most recent negative event you experienced in your life and ask yourself why it happened. Now consider the most recent positive occurrence and ask the same question. If you attribute the negative event to your own stupidity or to the dark cloud that always seems to hover overhead, you are leaning toward the pessimistic side of life. If you chalk up the positive event to a stroke of dumb luck that probably won't happen again, you are also displaying a pessimistic nature.

Psychologists have a more complex gauge for where people

stand on the optimism/pessimism scale. It's called explanatory style. As defined by Martin Seligman, Ph.D., of the University of Pennsylvania in Philadelphia, the pioneer in the field, explanatory style is your own unique way of defining and interpreting what happens to you: how you interpret, assess, and perceive the world. It's composed of three very specific decisions that you make in your mind about whatever happens to you:

◆ Is the incident your fault? Or is it the fault of others? If you blame yourself, you have an internal orientation; if you blame others, you have an external orientation.
◆ Is the cause temporary or will it linger in your mind? If you see repercussions as temporary, psychologists call this dimension unstable; if you let them linger, that's stable dimension.
◆ Does the cause affect one aspect of your life or many aspects? This is referred to among experts as specific vs. global.

People can blend these tendencies and fall anywhere on the continuum between the two extremes, but pessimists generally tend to explain negative events in an internal, stable, and global pattern. In other words, when something bad happens, they blame themselves, expect that the reason will linger for quite some time, and believe the event will affect many parts of their lives. Optimists, on the other hand, are essentially the opposite. They don't blame themselves, and they expect the consequences to be minor and of short duration; they also don't let it affect other parts of their lives.

To better understand explanatory style, let's pay another visit to Bob and Ellen and see how each reacts to failing an excruciatingly difficult midterm exam in biochemistry.

Even before the professor hands her the bad news, Ellen is convinced that she performed poorly. Her pessimism is confirmed when she receives her results. "See?" she says to herself. "I really am stupid." This response is clearly an internal answer. Lack of intellectual muster also is pretty stable and unlikely to change anytime soon. In fact, the test results reinforced the impression. Finally, the belief that she is stupid will no doubt affect many other areas of her life—a global response.

Now Bob, convinced from the outset that he aced the exam, gets his results (and his head) handed to him on a platter. After the brief initial shock, he suddenly recognizes that this was an entirely unfair test, an external response that removes the whole burden of blame from his shoulders. We've repeatedly seen students expend a tremendous amount of energy to prove that test questions were unfair or ambiguous, searching diligently for any explanation other than their own behavior (or lack of it).

Bob's belief that this particular test was unfair doesn't lead him to conclude that all tests are unfair, so here he falls on the unstable side of the style gauge. Lastly, one blatantly unjust biochemistry midterm doesn't mean much in the grand scheme of things—clearly, a specific answer.

After class, Ellen gets a headache and stays home in bed for 2 days. Bob all but forgets about his failing grade and spends the weekend skiing.

Pessimistic Predilections, Pessimistic Predictions

There's a solid mind-body explanation for Bob's and Ellen's contrasting reactions. Compared with their more optimistic counterparts, pessimists end up being sick more days in any given month, and they go to the doctor more frequently in any given year. So say the conclusions of a study from another pioneer in the field of explanatory style and health, Christopher Peterson, Ph.D., of the University of Michigan, Ann Arbor, who co-devised what has become the predominant determinant of explanatory style, the Attributional Style Questionnaire (ASQ).

Whether you are an optimist or pessimist determines not only your short-term health but your health decades later. Way back in the 1940s, researchers asked a group of Harvard graduates to answer a battery of questions. Some three decades later, Dr. Peterson, Dr. Seligman, and George Vaillant, M.D., of Dartmouth Medical School in Hanover, New Hampshire, took a look at the original data scored it for optimism or pessimism, and plotted the status of the study participants' health every 5 years until the original participants turned 60.

At ages 30, 35, and 40, no health discrepancies emerged between optimists and pessimists. Between ages 40 and 45, though, an interesting pattern did begin to manifest itself: The pessimists weren't quite as healthy as the optimists. They generally had more health problems, both major and minor. The relationship fell off a bit after the age of 45, for reasons the research trio could not explain. Nonetheless, the study's results stand as a powerful piece of evidence that how you perceive the world in your early 20s influences your health in your mid 40s.

What physiological and immunological mechanisms are at work here? Unfortunately, no one has a definitive answer. We do, however, have some clues. Pessimists have lower T cell ratios than optimists, according to work by Dr. Seligman and colleague Leslie Kamen-Siegel, Ph.D. Specifically, optimists have a higher ratio of helper T cells to suppressor T cells, a common measurement of the immune system's competence.

Our Study

The fact that pessimistic students in Dr. Peterson's study got colds and the flu more frequently suggested to us that IgA was involved, given that low IgA levels correlate with getting sick. We decided to test the proposition. The results surprised us.

In 1999, we gave the ASQ to 116 students at Wilkes University in Wilkes-Barre, Pennsylvania. While they answered questions, we took saliva samples to check for the presence of IgA. No relationship existed between either the overall scores and IgA nor between the optimism score and IgA. The more pessimistic they were or the more hopeless they felt, however, the lower their IgA levels. We didn't follow the students over the course of the year to see who got sick and who didn't; we just took a snapshot. But our results mesh beautifully with Dr. Peterson's findings that pessimists get colds and the flu more frequently than do optimists.

Why would a dark outlook on life influence health? Perhaps pessimism and hopelessness cause IgA levels to drop. Perhaps pessimists feel more stress, and its attendant immune effects, as they wait for disaster to strike. Maybe they just cannot sit back, relax, and enjoy life. Maybe it's a combination. Maybe it's something that science has yet to identify. What's clear, though, is that the worse you feel about yourself and the worse your outlook on life, the worse your health will be. For reasons mostly unknown, an optimist is healthier than a pessimist.

Down in the Dumps: Depressed Mood, Suppressed Health

Back when we didn't have doctors to give us shots, scribble out prescriptions, and advise us to slow down and get plenty of rest, we needed something that forced us to conserve energy and fight off illnesses. Otherwise, none of us would be here right now. That's what really gave birth to the blues.

True, it seems odd, but low moods and certain forms of depression actually may possess some sort of survival advantage. As mentioned in the previous chapter, depression is associated with many of the same changes that the presence of a microorganism produces physically—symptoms too numerous to chalk up to coincidence. Even a weird symptom like loss of appetite makes sense.

Slowing AIDS by Massaging Mood?

In considering damage to the body's natural defenses, you can't get more insidious than AIDS—acquired immunodeficiency syndrome. Among those infected with the human immunodeficiency virus (HIV), victims who possess brighter dispositions have better immune system activity.

People with AIDS have greater numbers of helper T cells in their bodies if they suffer less tension and anxiety and if they display less depression, dejection, fatigue, lethargy, anger, and hostility, according to one small 5-week study of 18 AIDS-afflicted people.

This is no small feat. HIV specifically targets these antibody-stimulating cells, also called CD4 cells. The virus attacks them directly. The best measure of the disease's progression is a decline in CD4 numbers. The more depressed the study participants were, the less vigor they felt, the more fear they experienced, and the less they were able to laugh. All of those characteristics corresponded with a higher level of the antigen called P24 that indicates the activation of HIV.

According to a related study, those who more frequently declined to do things just to please other people had higher levels of cytotoxic T (CD8) cells, virucidal cells, and natural killer cells. They felt less tension, less anxiety, and less fatigue. Those who exercised regularly and pampered themselves more also had higher measurements of natural killer cells.

Disease-producing bugs need iron from blood plasma to reproduce, and we get plasma iron only from food. (That's why you're supposed to starve a cold.)

As with stress (which, as we explain in chapter 3, also mimics in many physiological ways the body's reaction to an infection, injury, or illness), this is a lifesaving asset in the short term but a health killer if prolonged and unresolved. The parallel becomes even stronger when you realize that prolonged stress can lead headfirst into depression.

AIDS patients who were able to express emotions while reliving memories had more natural killer cells with a better ability to destroy viruses. And they lived longer than their more bottled-up counterparts.

Other studies verify some of these findings; a few others don't. One corroborative experiment, performed over 5 years, showed that depressed HIV-positive gay men had a steeper decline in helper T cells than their nondepressed counterparts. Another 5-year study of HIV-positive people discovered that those who lacked emotional support suffered from a greater fall in helper T cell counts over the course of their disease.

The fighting spirit lengthened lives by some 9 months, according to yet another study of HIV-positive gay men. Those who refused to accept the disease and its consequences lived longer than those who realistically resigned themselves to their fates.

One experiment throws a monkey wrench into the mechanism of general agreement that disposition and mood slow the progression of AIDS and affect various immunological measurements. It found no association at all between temperament or disposition and certain immune factors among people infected by HIV who had yet to progress to full-blown AIDS.

Why? We're not sure, but it seems that perhaps psychological dynamics influence immunity at different stages of the disease's progression.

Infected by Depression?

So close is the apparent connection between germs running rampant in your body and low mood that some forms of depression may have to be reclassified as infectious diseases. To explain the hypothesis, we have to look at a mounting body of evidence that's too compelling to ignore.

Remember the pro-inflammatory cytokines? A subset of immune activators (whose members include interleukin-1, interleukin-6, and tumor necrosis factor, or TNF), they're part of the primary phone lines that your immune system and your nervous system use to talk to each other. Cytokines tell the immune system to turn itself on and to get to work when you get an infection. As such, they're generally good to have around, but again, to return to a frequent theme in this book, only in moderation. Their presence in higher-than-normal numbers coincides with depression.

◆ Research demonstrates that both exposure to an infection-causing bug and administration of either of two cytokines (interleukin-1 beta, or interleukin-6) produce the same effects on the brain, namely, alterations of certain neurotransmitter levels that mimic the ones seen in the brains of depressed people. Antidepressant medications, including both tricyclic antidepressants (Elavil) and serotonin-selective reuptake inhibitors (Prozac and Zoloft) correct these neurotransmitter imbalances. Almost precisely when the neurotransmitter imbalance is normalized and relief from depression is experienced (usually about a month after starting to take the drug), cytokine counts drop dramatically.

◆ As five different studies, conducted by various researchers between 1987 and 1995, show, administering certain cytokines not only alters neurochemistry but it actually makes people feel depressed and stressed. They also find it more difficult to think clearly and flexibly, and they show a greater concern about their bodies.

◆ People with allergies and such autoimmune disorders as multiple sclerosis, rheumatoid arthritis, and systemic lupus erythematosus (all are conditions in which the immune system goes haywire) have higher cytokine levels in their bodies. They also have a higher incidence of depressive disorders. Chicken or egg? It could be either, or it could be both. (See "The Parallel Universe of Autoimmune Diseases" on page 44.)

◆ One of the most significant signs of depression—a general inability to experience pleasure, which experts call anhedonia—

overtakes rats that are given cytokine-generating substances. How do the rodents show that they're not happy? They don't frown or furrow their brows, nor do they sit dejectedly in a corner with their paws crossed over their chests. Instead, they lose their taste for sugary foods.

A normal, healthy rat has a tremendous sweet tooth. Medicating these same rodents with either a tricyclic antidepressant (imipramine) or a serotonin-selective reuptake inhibitor (Prozac) restores their fondness for sweets.

◆ In the winter, our bodies produce higher amounts of two cytokines, interferon alpha and interferon gamma. Shorter days, longer nights, and lack of natural light also are thought to be responsible for the wintertime blues known as seasonal affective disorder (SAD). Is the dearth of sun related to the surge of cytokines? Perhaps. We'll address light therapy a little more in chapter 8.

While we've focused on elevated cytokines, many other aspects of the immune system also lag as depressive mood rises. Depressed people have lower measurements of B lymphocytes, T lymphocytes, and helper T cells, as well as a poor inflammatory response. Depressed people also have fewer natural killer cells swimming around in their bodies, and those fewer assassins do a lot less work.

Stressed, Depressed

Cytokines figure prominently into the depression equation, but what's at work here? Science isn't sure. We don't know why moderate numbers of cytokines are beneficial or why an overload is detrimental. We don't know if the neurotransmitter imbalances cause the excessive cytokine secretion or if the higher cytokine counts disturb brain chemistry. We're not even sure how antidepressant drugs truly brighten mood. Do they work by reestablishing a better brain chemical balance, by lowering cytokines, or by both means?

The Parallel Universe of Autoimmune Diseases

Rheumatoid arthritis, we all know, is a joint disease. Multiple sclerosis is a disease of the nerves that control our muscles. They are also autoimmune disorders, though, and personality traits and mood states have been implicated in both.

As any science-fiction fan knows, a parallel universe is a kind of alternative reality to the "real" world in which people look the same but behave and act in drastically different, often opposite, ways. In movies and galaxy-cruising books, it's all imaginative fantasy, of course. But in health, autoimmune diseases represent a real-life alternative universe.

In this topsy-turvy world, the immune system isn't your internal defender against illness. It's your worst enemy and constant attacker, going into overdrive and confusing your body's own cells as foreign invaders that must be eradicated.

Given the thrust of this book, you might think that people with autoimmune diseases would be better off if their lives were filled with stress and pessimism and completely devoid of pleasure. Not so in this upside-down place. When you have rheumatoid arthritis, lupus, or another autoimmune disorder, the worse your disposition and frame of mind, the more destructive your immune system.

Let's look at a couple of studies that illustrate the curious, contradictory goings-on.

Complicating matters further are the machinations of another culprit, stress, which appears to be aiding and abetting in this emotional crime. The appearance of pro-inflammatory cytokines prompts the body to secrete cortisol, a stress hormone among whose myriad functions is to inhibit the further release of cytokines. At least that's how the system works if you are mentally healthy. If you are depressed, the automatic shutoff malfunctions. Cortisol fails to shut off the cytokine se-

Arthritis. Learning to cope with psychological problems seems to hit arthritis right at the heart of the problem, not in the immune system generally. People who saw a therapist for their various emotional woes, a study reveals, didn't necessarily have better blood measurements of immune system markers, but they did have less joint impairment and fewer signs of joint inflammation. Joint impairment varies right along with the immune system's inflammatory response. The lower the immune response, the better you control arthritis.

Your own perception of how well you cope (particularly with pain) predicts how well you do against rheumatic aches and discomfort. People who are better at coping, one study shows, have higher blood readings of suppressor T cells, which turn off marauding immune cells. For an autoimmune disease, the more suppressor T cells you have, the less joint pain you will experience.

Multiple sclerosis (MS). In this autoimmune dysfunction, the immune system directs its destructive attention to the delicate insulation, called the myelin sheath, covering the nerves that control our muscles. The emotional immune-related implications of this disease haven't been researched adequately, but a 1988 study found that highly anxious people with MS and depressive tendencies had higher numbers of helper T cells in their blood than their less-anxious, optimistic counterparts. Again, these immune cells are critical for an aggressive immune response, so if you have MS, the more helper T cells you have, presumably, the worse your disease.

cretion. The continued cytokine presence sparks the continued release of cortisol, which still doesn't turn off the cytokine spigot. It becomes a vicious cycle that fuels the dual fires of both stress and depression.

You don't have to be clinically depressed to suffer the health consequences of injured immunity. Down moods shy of a textbook definition of depression also disrupt immune activity. The effects aren't quite so dramatic, but they're still real and consequential.

Even daily or hourly mood shifts sway immunity, as researchers from the State University of New York at Stony Brook found in a 1987 study of university students. When you're feeling good about life, you have significantly higher levels of IgA, studies show, and you teem with T lymphocytes. When you are upset, angry or moody, even for a little while, your IgA drops markedly and your T lymphocytes slow to a crawl. For however long you pout and feel sorry for yourself, your defenses are down to some degree.

As if all this weren't depressing enough, a 1999 study showed that depressed people typically don't eat well, don't sleep well, and don't move around much. They're more likely to smoke and more likely to abuse alcohol and drugs. The bad habits compound the problem.

There is a flip side to this ominous, dark cloud: Pleasure. The more fun you insert into your life, the less depressed you'll be and the healthier you'll become. For instance, one long-term study demonstrated that the immune system's natural killer-cell activity picks up once depression is overcome successfully.

Personality Traits and Health States

Character traits also make a huge difference in how healthy you are. Let's look at several, including how you vent anger and other strong emotions, how controlling you are, and how helpless or hopeless you feel.

Healthy Venting of Emotions

A short fuse is a shortcut to an early coronary, right? Time and again, research demonstrates that hostile people who are quick to blow a gasket are setting themselves up for a heart attack.

Yes, hostility is a major contributing factor to your risk of high blood pressure, heart disease, other illnesses, and death. What's equally true, though, is that the inability to express feelings, particularly about negatively charged subjects, also is unhealthy, especially for the immune system.

The key is how you do it. Fiery, aggressive venting is as bad for your immune strength as is keeping the hostility pent up inside. Assertive yet tactful and rational venting, though, helps keep the immune system running smoothly on all cylinders.

The mechanisms behind how hostility and venting influence immunity aren't crystal clear. In the mid 1980s, one of us sought to determine the association between IgA levels and the coronary-prone type A personality, a large component of which is hostility. We found no significant relationship. Other work, though, has suggested that something is going on.

In several studies, scientists engaged people in one of two written discussions: either an innocuous, emotionally empty talk or a more highly charged conversation in which they had to divulge emotion-laden information about themselves. As the participants vented, over time scientists took various immune system measurements. Compared with the people who restrained from venting, those able to display higher levels of feelings turned out to have greater lymphocyte proliferation and bettter specific antibody responses.

A good number of studies confirm a higher risk of cancer (and a worse prognosis) for the type C personality (see "The Cancer Connection" on page 48). This is the person who outwardly appears to be pleasant and claims to be free of hostility, distress, fatigue, and a sense of helplessness but who actually is seething with dammed-up emotions. Such people often simply accept their fates—and their illnesses.

Other experiments support the idea that your immune system benefits when you let emotions out rather than keeping them bottled up. People able to evoke emotions and reveal negative feelings when asked to recall a traumatic experience pay fewer visits to the doctor's office and have better-functioning immune systems, according to a

The Cancer Connection

If you've been diagnosed with cancer, you cannot help but be upset, frightened, angry, anxious, stressed, depressed, and decidedly pessimistic. One-third of all women and half of all men in the United States are going to get a malignant tumor somewhere in their bodies at some point in their lives, according to statistics from the American Cancer Society.

The research is mixed, but we suggest you fight rather than resign yourself to the disease. The better you handle the diagnosis and the better you grapple with your life after the diagnosis, the better your immune system will function.

Some long-term research concludes that depression predicts the later development and course of cancer. A 17-year study of 2,020 Western Electric employees, for example, calculated a twofold increase in the odds of dying from cancer among people who have depressive tendencies. While other researchers have identified no such association, the overall evidence is powerful enough to label depression a bona fide risk factor for cancer.

Some studies suggest that depression wounds your cells' ability to heal DNA, an impairment that would increase your vulnerability to carcinogens. Other research speculates that being depressed some time before a cancer diagnosis stems from the immune system's disturbance of a brain chemical (serotonin) related to low mood.

1987 study at Ohio State University in Columbus. They also stand a better chance of living longer and more comfortably if they have either AIDS or cancer (see "Slowing AIDS by Massaging Mood?" on page 40 and "The Cancer Connection").

Even if you've previously suppressed emotions, you can expect to enjoy a greater surge of immune system protection if you learn to vent bottled-up feelings. In follow-up studies, the venters' immune systems responded better to a hepatitis B vaccination than did those who continued to suppress how they really felt.

A final piece of evidence that releasing emotion is good and

Once the tumor is active, your disposition and emotional makeup seem to play a role in how bad the disease becomes and how successfully your body battles it. In a study of people with malignant melanoma, those who didn't express their emotions very well had thicker, more rapidly growing tumors and far fewer lymphocytes traveling to the cancerous site.

A different study comparing people with melanoma to people with cardiovascular disease found that the cancer patients displayed greater psychological and physiological responses to distressing occurrences, even though they claimed to feel far milder reactions. Another study of people with cancer who claimed to be calm, cool, and well-adjusted to the disease but who benefited from little social support and felt tired all the time also showed lower levels of natural killer cell activity. Much research on people with a repressive style of coping has documented disruptions in other aspects of immune effectiveness.

On the upside, the better you feel and the happier you are can figure in to how long you are going to live. Expressing more joy was the one psychological variable that stood out as a predictor of survival in a 7-year study of 36 women with breast cancer. We recommend that you seek out the pleasurable things in life no matter how difficult the diagnosis.

that suppressing it is bad: People were asked either to refrain from expressing emotional thoughts or to fully vent as they wrote brief essays. Those who opened up had better immune activity, showing greater numbers of circulating lymphocytes and helper T cells.

Inventing the Esteem Engine

In what was once a regular feature on the TV show *Saturday Night Live*, Al Franken, portraying Stuart Smalley, parodied the Hallmark Cards version of self-esteem. Franken poked fun at love-yourself pop psychology, but there's a grain of truth in his biting humor: The better you think of yourself, the better off you are and the healthier you are.

Experts aren't sure about how the concept of self-esteem fits into a person's overall personality profile. It's related, to at least some extent, to whether you are an optimist or a pessimist; it probably figures in to how negative you are (or aren't) and your tendency to lapse into blue moods. Nevertheless, while the evidence is not overwhelming, intriguing indications suggest that the higher your sense of self-esteem, the stronger your immune system. Here are three examples.

◆ A 1999 study showed that people with low self-esteem had poorer responses to rubella vaccinations than those with higher self-esteem, a difference that didn't manifest itself if any of the people already had rubella antibodies in their bloodstreams.

◆ Several 1999 studies at McGill University in Montreal demonstrated that self-esteem predicts quality of life and disease progression among women with systemic lupus erythematosus, an autoimmune disorder characterized by, among other problems, organ damage, lung inflammation, connective tissue disorders, and skin rashes. The women with low self-esteem had a greater degree of organ damage and a higher level of psychological distress.

◆ Among people with the jaw pain of temporomandibular disorder (TMD), the lower their self-esteem, the worse their immune systems operated, according to a study from Columbia University in New York.

Our Study

Our interest piqued, we decided to examine the relationship between self-esteem and our favorite immune antibody, IgA. As before, we had study participants deposit saliva in a cup, but this time we gave them a questionnaire called the Coopersmith Self-Esteem

Inventory. (This was a small pilot study reporting only preliminary results.) The participants with higher self-esteem had higher levels of IgA in their saliva.

Why? Again, we're not sure. Apparently, possessing a good sense of self is like being optimistic: It boosts your immune health. Which comes first? Yet again, no one really knows, but the two probably go hand in hand. Optimists probably have decent self-esteem, and people with a high sense of self-esteem are probably more optimistic. The bottom line, though, remains the same: Feeling good about yourself improves your health.

Don't Go Along to Get Along

If you want to do something to make someone happy, you probably can expect both an emotional and an immunological reward. But what if you grudgingly do something you really don't want to do? Emotionally, you can probably put up with performing the favor without too much distress. Your immune system, though, isn't so tolerant.

If you go along just to please another person, your immune system is going to suffer, according to a couple of 1987 studies. Those who voiced their reluctance and refused to go with the group had better-functioning immune systems, with higher levels of cytotoxic T (CD8) cells, virucidal cells, and natural killer cells.

What does this mean? No one knows for sure, but the best guess is that doing something that you really don't want to do elicits anger and frustration, two emotions that aren't going to do a lot of good to your immune system.

Power Tripping

They're go-getters, with high ambitions and perhaps an even higher need for control. But, when inhibited or prevented from expressing their aggressive tendencies directly, people with a strong power motivation are setting themselves up for a higher risk of disease.

A Woman's Outlook

Postpartum depression upsets the lives of many new mothers who could be teeming with delight because of their little bundles of joy. What's upsetting them so? Maybe the party-crashing presence of a group of immune activators called pro-inflammatory cytokines, the main means by which the nervous system communicates with the immune system. Cytokine secretion soars during childbirth and can influence how you feel well after, according to a 1993 study.

Whether pregnant, in labor, or child-free, women generally have a higher degree of immune activation than men. They're also twice as likely than men to experience a depressive disorder. Estrogen apparently tends to make a woman's immune system more sensitive and more likely to react, whether for the good or the bad. The implications are unclear, as are the reasons. Lamentably, studies on gender differences in this respect are scarce.

College students classified as high in power motivation, for instance, tend to have lower levels of IgA than their peers and tend to get sick more frequently, one study found. Another, this one conducted during academic test time, noticed that IgA measurements of power-people who couldn't exercise control fell during and even well after the exams, while those of their less power hungry counterparts soon returned to normal levels. Students whose power motivation was stronger than their desire to interact with others, yet another experiment concluded, possessed lower IgA almost 2 hours after taking a test than those who preferred to hang out with friends rather than flex their control muscles.

Helplessly Hopeless

Being unable to exert control and power is bad for your immune system, but so is resigning yourself to helplessness and hopelessness.

Consider the case of Jane, who's suffering from depression and trying to overcome it through weekly visits to a psychologist.

On an especially gloomy day in Jane's mind, the therapist suggests that she, a real clotheshorse in better times, go to the mall and buy a new outfit. Depression, the doctor knows, saps people of their initiative, and doing something—anything—is going to boost their spirits. Inactivity, moreover, is the one characteristic of mood most likely to wound immune activity.

Easier said than done. Jane resists. First, she says it's her husband's day for the car. But he, a retiree, doesn't plan to go anywhere, the therapist soon learns. This would be an excellent opportunity for Jane to assert herself and, simply by doing so, perk up her immune activity. She again demurs. What about taking the bus? Jane doesn't know the schedule. Even when the therapist gives her the bus times, she expresses reluctance to go to the mall. She even says that despite the lavish, opulent shops there, she probably wouldn't find anything worth buying.

This is classic excuse-making by someone who feels that she has no control over her life. Jane's attitude is perpetuating her depression. She obviously feels helpless. She also feels hopeless, which, as psychologists define it, is the belief that helplessness will persist. Jane needs to understand that she must exercise some control because the consequences of helplessness and hopelessness can be terribly destructive to the immune system.

Immune analyses of people who display hopelessness reveal myriad changes in their natural killer cells, cytotoxic T cells, and IgA. The overall impact of feeling hopeless is devastating. For instance, our 1999 study of Wilkes University students found that the more hopeless a student felt, the lower his or her IgA measurements.

Animal experiments also demonstrate the impact of helplessness on immune function. In 1978, researchers from Carleton University in Ottawa, Canada, implanted cancerous tumors in three groups of lab rats. They then subjected two of the groups to electrical shocks. (The jolts are strong enough to cause a stress response, but they're otherwise mild and inflict no damage.) Rats in one of the two groups could turn off the shock by pressing a lever; those in the other group could not.

The rats that weren't jolted had the least extent of tumor growth. Both groups exposed to the electric shocks experienced a higher incidence of tumor growth, although the incidence of cancer in the group able to shut off the shock was significantly lower than in the helpless group.

In a similar experiment, conducted at Rockefeller University in New York City in 1972, two of three groups of rats again were given electrical shocks. This time, the difference was that for one group, a light flashed in their cages just before and during the jolt. Rats in both shocked groups later developed more gastric ulcers, but those that saw the pre-shock light ended up better off; they didn't have as many stomach sores.

Why? As the Rockefeller researchers speculated, the flashing light allowed the rats to predict the assault. They came to learn that when the light was off, they could relax. The other rats suffered from chronic, continuous anxiety and stress; they could never relax or let their guards down because their electrical assaults were entirely unpredictable and random.

The moral? Even if the stressor and the reaction are the same for two people, introducing a little bit of predictability and control could make a difference on the ultimate impact on health.

Now, back to Jane. In the end, the psychologist, as part of her therapy, required her to go to the mall, exercise some independence and control, have a bit of fun, and buy a new dress. The shopping trip rebuffed her why-bother attitude. She enjoyed herself, found a great outfit, and, as a result, felt less depressed.

Getting Connected . . .
with a More Positive Attitude

Being negative, feeling helpless, stopping up emotions, and generally not seeing the sunny side of life all help lead to anhedonia, the inability to appreciate the pleasures of life. Anhedonia is one of the two principal telltale signs of depression; actual depressed mood is the other. When even things you used to enjoy—seeing a movie, going to parties, listening to music, savoring food—are no longer fun, you're headed down a path that's far more than colorless and dull. And as most of the evidence indicates, if you're not having any fun, you're probably less physically healthy than you could be. The more pessimistic, hopeless, vulnerable, and depressed you are, the more you need to inject a little fun into your life.

The first step in plugging into the Immunity-Pleasure Connection involves making some significant attitude adjustments. Some tricks of the trade will facilitate this fine-tuning.

Just do it. Even if you don't feel like getting off the couch, taking a shower, and going to the theater to see that movie you thought might be good, do it anyway. Go to that party. Run down to the music store and buy the new CD by your favorite band. Drag yourself to the gym.

Most of us think that attitude must change before behavior changes. That's true, but the inverse works too. If you force yourself to behave in a way that's out of synch with how you actually feel, your brain won't long be able to tolerate the incongruity. It'll change your attitude to come into accordance with your behavior. In psychological lingo, the term is *cognitive dissonance*. A dramatic example is the Stockholm Effect, in which hostages develop sympathy for or an affinity with their captors because they've been trying, in an effort to survive the ordeal, to comply with and please their abductors.

Avoid secondhand pessimism. Minimize the time you spend with complainers, doubters, and other pessimists. Think of negativity as the emotional equivalent of a room filled with cigarette smoke. Pessimism is a psychologically contagious disease.

Get it off your chest. This is crucial. Vent repressed, emotionally charged feelings. At least once a week, visit with or call a different friend or family member and talk about something that's been bothering you. Cycle through your list of confidantes and then start all over again. If they know that their listening helps you, the sense of reward that they derive will benefit their immune systems too. And it might not be a bad idea to meet over a drink or two. According to a study conducted at Harvard on longevity, in moderation alcohol can facilitate disclosure and break down your resistance to opening up, which will benefit your well-being. (But remember that beyond moderation alcohol has the opposite effect.)

Let go of hostility (but don't assault). If you're ticked off at somebody or if someone puts you in a position that frustrates or irritates you, say so, albeit in a tactful manner. Research shows that blowing up at the transgressor will not truly help you dispense with your anger. Five minutes after venting your frustration in this manner, you are likely to be even more angry, champing at the bit to let 'em have it all over again.

So, do indeed communicate your feelings. Be assertive, open, and honest. But also be calm, considerate, tactful, and polite.

Howl at the moon. What about a private temper tantrum? Well, it's best to directly address the object of your anger, but stomping around the house and screaming at the ceiling might help.

Grin—it helps you bear it. Whether or not you have reason to do so, smile frequently. The nerves connected to your face's smile muscles project right into parts of the brain that help determine mood. Send a signal to your brain that you're happy, and voilà! You *are* happy (and so is your immune system). Sure, it's a trick, but it's one that works. It's also a twist on the old Descartes dictum, "I think, therefore I am." Descartes, like many of the rest of us, surely had a mother who also advised, "Smile, you'll feel better."

Give yourself a round of applause. If something good happens, give yourself the credit you deserve. Make a big deal out of it. When something unfortunate occurs, don't dwell on it. Consider the circumstances surrounding it and assess your responsibility. Then put it behind you and move on. Don't bad-mouth yourself. Many people engage in highly negative dialogues with themselves: "I'm stupid"; "I'm unattractive"; "I can't do anything right." This insulting, degrading self-talk leads to everything from pessimism and poor self-esteem to depression. Stop putting yourself down. Develop a list of positive assertions about yourself and refer to it every time you start to put yourself down. Use it often and think well of yourself. Self-esteem is good for the immune system. You don't have to be outstanding; just perceive yourself to be.

Tell yourself a little white lie. In assessing your strengths, you don't even have to be completely accurate or honest. In fact, sometimes the worst thing you can do is be honest. It turns out that little white lies are little white pills that strengthen your immune system and enable you to be healthier.

The more accurately you perceive reality, the more likely you are going to be depressed, according to Dr. Seligman. We're not going to advocate that you become a pathological liar, but we will excuse an occasional fib that lets you get on with life and allows you to be healthier. In the name of deluding disease, sometimes you should delude yourself. Give yourself the benefit of the doubt regarding the fairness of the test you failed or job interview that didn't go well.

Get on a winning streak. Nothing succeeds like success, so set yourself up for a string of victories. Put yourself into situations that can have only positive outcomes. As you experience success, you'll begin to perceive yourself as successful. Your perception of yourself then dictates your behavior. For example, if you have a few positive social experiences, such as having a great time at a party or finding new friends by going to the gym, you'll tend to see the world as a warm, friendly place, and you'll tend to interact with your world in a warmer, more friendly manner. People around you will respond to you in accordance with your behavior, and your behavior will inevitably become even warmer and more friendly.

Plan to prolong pleasure. If you do something spontaneously on Saturday night, you and your immune system will enjoy it, but only on Saturday night. If you plan the activity on Thursday, though, you'll look forward to the enjoyment all day Thursday, all day Friday, and all day Saturday. Anticipation helps determine mood. Anticipating a negative event provokes anxiety and, if continued long enough, depression. Anticipating a positive event, on the other hand, brightens your mood and attitude. Pleasure and anhedonia cannot coexist, so plan your fun and make the most of it.

As soon as you finish reading this chapter, put down the book and plan to do something fun 2 days from now. It doesn't have to be a major production; even a trivial activity will suffice. The event isn't important. What's important is the planning.

Be a fighter (but not a bully). Studies show that fighting for something and losing, even in situations where the odds seem insurmountable, helps prevent the kind of immune system slowdown suffered by subjects who give up.

But taking this attitude to the extreme, as bullies often do, can have the opposite effect. Harvard researcher David McClelland, Ph.D., found that people in a sample with a strong power motive and high stress had lower IgA levels and the highest frequency of illness.

Be a discloser (but not a complainer). Release negative emotion in appropriate ways with confidants. Describe situations and ask for advice, but don't spout and moan. You don't necessarily have to take their advice, but asking for it will lift their self-esteem, and you'll have a willing audience for your immunoenhancement.

Be humorous and quick to laugh. Humor benefits more than just the immune system, and amusing others amuses us.

Be in control. It's amazing how much of our lives we can control if we think about it. This is good. Choose these things to focus on. Even if a situation is bad, exert some control. Don't wait all day for a confrontational phone call. Make the call now at 9:00 A.M. instead of receiving it at 1:00 P.M. and suffering 4 hours of anticipatory anxiety. Your immune system hates this.

Be optimistic. Don't focus on the negative things that you have no control over. At any point in time, 90 percent of our lives may be a mess and uncontrollable. Focus 90 percent of your time on the 10 percent that you can control for positive effects, and you'll do well 90 percent of the time.

Be assertive (but not aggressive). Be that person who says no to a request in such a way that the requestor walks away feeling that he was done a favor. Do this by offering better alternatives or creating humor to diffuse conflict.

Don't stay anxious or sad. Use negative states as alarm clocks. Wake up and do something about them immediately. Don't let them change from states to traits.

Chapter 3

The Stress Mess

FIGHT, FLIGHT, AND THE IMMUNITY-PLEASURE CONNECTION

Reality is the leading cause of stress
amongst those in touch with it.
—Jane Wagner, writer, humorist, and director;
and Lily Tomlin, comedienne and actor

The alarm didn't go off, and now you're late for work—again. No sympathy and assistance this time from your significant other, who's still chilly following the argument the night before about going to that party. No solace on the ride to work, either. You hit the rush hour at its peak, and the car makes strange knocking noises the whole time. Nothing interesting on the radio, either. Bad songs, bad talk, bad news that you don't want to hear.

After a typically harrowing day at work, you get stuck in a long queue at the grocery store's curiously named express line. The cashier obviously is a kid with only a day's worth of on-the-job experience, and someone six customers in front of you is writing a check for a $3 purchase. A dispute over ID ensues. You roll your eyes and scan the tabloid headlines again. Another shopper in front of you has just placed 20 items on the conveyor belt (you counted them three times while waiting) in a line reserved for a maximum of 10.

Yes, another one of those days, a day during which spontaneous combustion doesn't seem an unlikely possibility (or entirely unwelcome, for that matter).

Our lives are filled with such stressful episodes. In and of themselves, no one incident may be a killer, but both little irritants and major problems all add up and exact a cumulative price on your psyche and your health. In every way, stress is the absolute antithesis of pleasure. It jangles your nerves, juggles a whole host of your body's hormones, elevates your blood pressure, and makes your pulse race. It keeps you on edge, disturbs your sleep, disrupts your appetite, upsets your stomach, gives you a quite literal pain in the neck (or shoulders), and interferes with your enjoyment of life. It also weakens your immune system's ability to resist illness and disease. In short, the more stressful your life, the more likely you're going to get sick.

If you don't siphon off stress on a day-by-day basis, you're setting yourself up for problems somewhere down the road. It may not be today. It may not be tomorrow. It might be next week, and it almost certainly will be a couple of months from now. Stress quite literally could kill you in any number of ways. Counteracting the physiological and psychological damage of stress could very well restore your good health and literally save your life.

Pinning Down Stress

We all know what stress feels like, but what exactly is it? Simply put, it's what happens to the body when we perceive a threat, whether real or imagined, physical or psychological, that we're not sure we can successfully handle. Stress tends to lead to anxiety, which only leads to more stress. The more frequently you experience a certain stressor, the more likely you'll anxiously expect it and get stressed out, even if that stressor turns out to be nonexistent at a particular time. In other words, if you've fumed and fretted enough times in that express checkout, you may get stressed even when you push the buggy to the counter and you see that there's no one else in line.

So how do you know when the stress in your life has become chronic enough to pose a health problem? That is difficult to determine with any precision. Nature designed stress as a short-term response. Technically, therefore, anything that stressfully arouses the body for more than several minutes could be considered a chronic problem. Most experts, though, would define chronic stress as persisting for more than several weeks.

Stress damage is cumulative over time and across situations. No one stressful incident may cause a problem, but all the little episodes encountered over time add up and inflict the same devastating effects as one major, prolonged event. The fewer minor irritants you have in your life, the better off you're going to be. Similarly, the more you offset all of the irritants with pleasurable distractions, the less vulnerable you will be.

One of the psychological standards for assessing the health impact of stress, the Rahe Life Stress Scale, adds up stress-producing occurrences over an entire year in quantifying your stress level and the likelihood that it will impair your health (see "How Stressed Are You?" on page 76).

Fight, Flee, or Fry: Why We Get Stressed

Difficult as it may be to believe, the stress response actually is a wonderful survival mechanism. When we lived in caves and regularly confronted bears, beasts, and other physical threats, stress was a good thing, revving up and girding our bodies for brief battles against threats to our security and well-being. But today, we live in condominiums and confront predators of a different sort: sharks and snakes that wear ties, skirts, and supermarket smocks. Sure, we still could be mugged or attacked by an animal, but the nature of stressful encounters has changed over the past several thousand years far more quickly than our ability to adapt. Nowadays, most stress-evoking conflicts aren't physical. They're psychological. But your body can't really tell the difference between, say, a snarling, menacing saber-toothed tiger, an inconsiderate shopper with too many items in the express lane, and a TV that goes on the fritz while 50 friends are gathered in your living room to watch the Super Bowl. The body reacts the same way in each case.

That greatly limits options. You probably won't punch out the back-stabbing coworker. There's no point in running wildly from the grocery store with your arms flailing above your head. And you can't fix the TV by banging your fist on top of it.

The transformed nature of stress hinders our ability to recover from the physiological changes that we undergo. If you fight or flee, the exertion helps your physiology return to normal, which is why exercise is a good stress reducer. If you just put up and shut up with the stress, sit and seethe, or let it go unresolved for any length of time, the chemicals responsible for the physiological responses continue to churn inside you with rather adverse effects.

The Good Old Days

To better understand why we experience stress and why it's now a health problem, we need to travel thousands of years back in time, when our ancestors were club-carrying hunter-gatherers. Put yourself in their place. Life was hard, food often was scarce, and day-to-day living frequently involved great struggles to eat and avoid being eaten. Imagine a quite stressful confrontation with a poised-to-pounce saber-toothed tiger. You have two options: Fight the big beast *mano-a-gato*, or run like hell.

What possible physiological changes could your body undergo to help you avoid being a canapé for the killer cat? You could certainly use a little more strength in your throwing arm for some well-aimed, solidly hurled rocks or spears. You could benefit from some extra energy for fleeter feet. You also need keener senses and brain power to help you decide whether to fight, flee, or toss rocks behind you as you make a mad dash. To get out of this mess, you need a fully stoked mind and body. You need to be primed for the fight or flight of your life.

Gearing Up

The stress response allows you to gear up. A two-pronged physiological response, dubbed the fight-or-flight stress response by eminent Harvard physiologist Walter Cannon, M.D., evolved to help humans do just that. When a stressful encounter is perceived, the brain and body automatically coordinate a number of physiologic events, shunting more energy and resources to some systems while weakening or virtually shutting down others. (To see how your body orchestrates these changes, see "The Nervy Chemistry of Stress" on page 66.)

Cardiovascular system. At the expense of just about every other body system, your cardiovascular system receives an enormous boost from the stress response. Bloodflow increases to the heart and vital organs because they all need more oxygen. You're about to flee or fight, after all. At the same time, arteries constrict in the limbs, hands, and feet, reducing bloodflow to those spots to decrease the possibility of bleeding to death if injured. The net effect of these cardiovascular changes is a tremendous increase in blood pressure, a rapid quickening of pulse rate, and an increased demand on the heart muscle.

(continued on page 68)

The Nervy Chemistry of Stress

Three hormones secreted from your adrenal glands—cortisol, epinephrine, and norepinephrine—share the credit (or blame) for most of the changes that you experience when you're stressed. How your body releases them provides a biological explanation for the fact that you cannot be stressed and happily content at the same time.

Let's take a closer look under the hood and see what fuels your stress engine and what tosses a monkey wrench into your internal fun factory.

Hardwiring and Health

The adrenal glands, which sit atop your kidneys, are the source of the chemicals that make you feel frazzled and prevent you from having fun. They release their pleasure-constraining hormones through a complex network of nerves and battery of actions that requires a mini-lesson in neuroendocrine anatomy. We'll keep it simple.

The brain and spinal cord comprise our central nervous system. All the remaining neural wiring in our bodies attached to the brain and spinal cord is known collectively as the peripheral nervous system, which consists of two parts, the somatic and the autonomic. The somatic nervous system enables all of our willful, voluntary movements, such as flexing a muscle, moving our eyes, and blowing our noses. The autonomic nervous system is a separate set of circuitry that rules over all involuntary behavior. ("Autonomic" sounds like "automatic," and the two words essentially are synonymous.) It regulates respiration, digestion, heartbeat, and blood pressure. For our purposes here, the autonomic part of our circuitry determines if we're bested by stress or pleasurably content.

The autonomic nervous system itself consists of two branches, the sympathetic and the parasympathetic systems. Each operates via entirely different paths and releases entirely different chemicals that govern completely different and opposing physiological and emotional states. Let's break them down.

Good times. During unstressed periods, the parasympathetic nervous system runs the show, signaling certain nerves and releasing chemicals.

Bad times. Immediately upon your perception of stress, tension, anxiety, fear, and other negative states, the sympathetic nervous system jumps to the fore and suppresses the parasympathetic branch. From here on until you recover from whatever is bothering you, the sympathetic nervous system is in charge. It directly stimulates nerves to trigger the adrenal glands into releasing epinephrine and norepinephrine, which then initiate the whole fight-or-flight response.

Given the opposing nature of the two branches, the sympathetic and parasympathetic systems cannot be activated simultaneously. You cannot be stressed out and chilled out at the same time. While it's true that stress cranks up the sympathetic engine, the reverse also is true: Parasympathetic activity turns the sympathetic motor off and pulls the key out of the ignition. A high degree of activity in one system deactivates the other.

Longer-Term Logistics

The autonomic reaction and the release of epinephrine and norepinephrine represent your almost instantaneous physiological response to stress. Bringing up the rear a little later for slower-acting, longer-term duty and damage while stressed is another hormone from the adrenal glands: cortisol.

Cortisol is a major culprit in many of the physiological changes that you undergo when you're stressed out, particularly the elevation of blood sugar (that's why it is also known as a glucocorticoid). It also tames inflammation, suppresses immune system activity, and possibly kills brain cells. Its higher concentration in the stressed body is undeniable. We can get a rough indication of how stressed you are simply by measuring how much cortisol is in your blood or saliva.

Cortisol is secreted through a pathway called the hypothalamic-pituitary-adrenal (HPA) axis. What occurs is this: Upon recognizing something stressful, the hypothalamus releases a chemical called CRH that in turn tells the pituitary gland to release a substance called ACTH, which swims through the bloodstream and tells the adrenals to pump out cortisol. This chemical connection is indisputable. According to experiments conducted on both people and animals, if you block CRH, the entire chain of events is short-circuited. ACTH is not secreted, cortisol is not secreted, and the immune system functions normally.

Energy. To fuel the anticipated exertion, the body releases blood sugar (glucose) from tissue stores. Glucose is the body's prime source of energy. For additional energy, the body also releases stored fat into the bloodstream.

Mental faculties. More blood flows to the brain as well. You have to make snap decisions about whether to stand your ground or hightail it out of there.

Shutting Down

The extra energy and reallocation of resources comes at a cost to other bodily functions. Two in particular get short shrift.

Reproductive system. Thank the saber-toothed tiger and other nerve agitators for your inability to get "in the mood" when you're stressed out, anxious, or edgy. The reproductive system is very energy intensive, and nature has seen to it that sexual function is all but shut off to redirect energy elsewhere.

Immune system. How likely is it that you'll encounter a serious pathogen in the 60 seconds following your initial spotting of the big-fanged tiger? Not likely. Some of the enormous amount of energy necessary to fuel the highly complex group of cells, organs, and hormones that comprises the immune system is better directed elsewhere at this moment.

The reallocation of resources is of little consequence if the stressful episode is brief. And besides, the gearing down often leaves immune measurements within an acceptable, if somewhat low, range of "normal."

Pain perception. What if the saber-toothed tiger manages to chew off a chunk of your arm? The agony would certainly detract from your ability to enjoy life. To avoid this possibility, the body increases the secretion of pain-numbing endorphins and other natural opiates.

From Death to Taxes:
How Stress Knocks Down Defenses

Of all the physiological aspects of the stress response, a weakened immune system is the most serious, and the hardest to explain. Sure, you can get by for a while without the ability to become sexually aroused or without an acute sensitivity to pain. But the ability to fight off germs? Why would the body take such a chance? Science doesn't know for certain, and researchers are far from unanimous in their findings. Science is not even certain how dramatically stress weakens the immune system. Depending upon such variables as the nature of the stressor, its intensity, and its duration, some research finds that the reduction is slight. Other research concludes that the impact is devastating. Many studies show that the reduced activity may still be within a range considered normal.

Normal, however, is not ideal. Disputes over degree may be irrelevant, however, for even slight reductions in immunity can have serious consequences in fending off illness. What is beyond dispute scientifically, though, is that overwhelming evidence demonstrates that stress and the substances it causes to be secreted in the body negatively affect your ability to remain healthy. From immunoglobulin A (IgA) to natural killer-cell activity, almost any immune system component suffers a loss of strength in the presence of stress. We also know with almost absolute certainty that relieving tension and anxiety improves your ability to resist getting sick.

Any Way You Slice It

The number of stress-evoking events in life corresponds rather well to at least some lowering of the body's natural defenses. So strong is the association that you can expect any highly stressful occurrence—an IRS audit, being robbed by a thug in a dark alley, a flat tire on a busy highway, your suddenly independent teenager wanting to move to the other side of the country, getting laid off from work—to interfere with the optimal workings of your body's natural defenses. A continual series of minor stressors accomplishes the same thing, but the more traumatic the event, the greater and longer-lasting the immune wound. A study at the University of the Health Sciences in Bethesda, Maryland, showed that people who lived near Three Mile Island in Pennsylvania when the nuclear power plant there nearly melted down in 1979 showed impaired immune activity for years after the accident.

Death of a spouse nearly tops the list of most traumatically stressful events on the Rahe Scale, followed soon after by the figurative death of a marriage through divorce. The unpredictability and uncontrollability of such situations, along with the drastic change in daily routine and the loss of a longtime confidant, all come at an emotionally and physically high price. In virtually any way you choose to measure it, the immune systems of people coping with the death of a spouse, a separation, or a divorce show decided degrees of weakness, according to a number of studies by Ronald Glaser, Ph.D., and Janice Kiecolt-Glaser, Ph.D., a research duo at Ohio State University in Columbus. Recovery and getting back to "normal," both psychologically and immunologically, typically takes several years, the research duo concludes. (For more on how the stress of grief and separation disturb immune function, see chapter 5.)

No Coincidental Connection

Is the connection between stress and immunity a direct one? Apparently so. Animal experiments predominate in this area, because you cannot, ethically, deliberately expose people to pain or major peril. Still, using innovative ways to get around the problem, researchers have discerned direct connections between level of stress and degree of immune decrease.

Why the Weakening?

Even though it seems pretty clear that stress prevents your body from fighting off infections and illnesses, the question still remains: Why? It just doesn't make a whole lot of sense. Why would a so-called survival mechanism sabotage your chances of surviving?

Theories abound, but yet again, no one knows for sure. Yes, shunting energy stores to more important functions like fighting or fleeing makes sense—for momentary emergencies, as nature intended. But it still doesn't offer a full explanation. Why, even for a couple of minutes, risk getting an infection? Why bare your neck and leave yourself so vulnerable? Some experts say that the stress hormone cortisol's hindering of immune activity is like your foot pushing on the brake pedal of a car: The stress chemical slows an action that would otherwise build momentum and get out of control. People whose bodies cannot secrete cortisol do, in fact, have a higher risk for developing rheumatoid arthritis, asthma, multiple sclerosis, and other autoimmune afflictions, including Addison's disease, the adrenal gland dysfunction that plagued John F. Kennedy. Lesser secretions do not necessarily cause disease but do, apparently, cause problems.

Other experts liken stress to an infectious illness. That's not a bad analogy. Whether you are stressed out or whether you are infected by some unknown pathogen, the immune system reacts in basically the same way. In fact, researchers Steven Maier, Ph.D., and Linda Watkins, Ph.D., of the University of Colorado at Boulder, theorize that the stress response actually evolved out of and is largely the result of immune system activation. Whether you're infected or stressed, the innate immune system—the general, all-purpose defense system that we're all born with—comes into play. At the same time, what's termed *acquired immunity* takes a backseat and is deemphasized. Acquired immunity is how your immune system adapts to a very precise, specific bug. When you get a polio vaccine, for instance, your acquired immunity kicks into gear and learns how to defend you against that particular bug. Again, the emphasis on innate immunity at the expense of acquired immunity may be helpful in a momentary crisis but proves to be anything but beneficial when prolonged.

Some scientists give their study participants difficult math problems or almost-unsolveable anagrams. Others have compelled their human participants to make speeches before audiences. For instance, the more nervous you feel about making a presentation, according to a 1995 study of 19 women conducted by Karen Mathews, Ph.D., at the University of Pittsburgh School of Medicine, the more your immune system will weaken. As opposed to death being the number 1 stress inducer, delivering a public speech is the number 1 anxiety-producing fear among Americans. Remember, anxiety is the fearful anticipation of a future stress-evoking occurrence. In this regard, it's interesting to note that death is the number 2 fear, a fact that once prompted comic Jerry Seinfeld to quip that at a funeral, many people would rather be the person in the coffin than the person delivering the eulogy.

Nevertheless, whether agitated by stress or anxiety, your emotional state at the time you are infected with a pathogen makes all the difference, according to a uniquely valuable 1991 study by Sheldon Cohen, Ph.D., of Carnegie Mellon University in Pittsburgh. In his experiment, 394 people consented to being exposed to the rhinovirus that causes the common cold. Afterward, those who described themselves as "highly stressed" were twice as likely to develop cold symptoms as their low-stress counterparts. Every single one of them still had immune systems within "normal" and "healthy" ranges, but even slight stress-related immune weakness left them more susceptible to the virus.

As noted, scientifically assessing the impact of stress on immunity is extremely difficult. Researchers can gauge associations indirectly by asking questions and then taking measurements, but they generally cannot infect people, subject them to stress, and then wait to see who falls ill. Ethics aside, you are not likely to get many volunteers for such an experiment.

We are constantly exposed to untold numbers of bugs, yet we

don't always get sick. What spells the difference? Considerable research, including Dr. Cohen's study, clearly hints that stress suppresses immunity sufficiently enough to render us more vulnerable. And support for the contention that the longer the stress, the worse off you are comes from a follow-up study of 276 people that Dr. Cohen conducted in 1998. Intense but limited episodes of stress are not associated with getting a cold, he concluded. However, severe chronic stress extending for more than a month did correspond with more instances of the sniffles.

Animal experimentation backs up the results seen with people. When you expose rats to such stress inducers as electrical shocks or the mammalian equivalent of being accosted by bullies, the rodents' immune systems display distinct signs of weakening, according to a number of impressive studies by two top psychoneuroimmunology researchers from the University of Colorado at Boulder, Steven Maier, Ph.D., and Linda Watkins, Ph.D. In one experiment, the scientists injected a bunch of rats with a substance called KLH, an innocent protein that, because it's a foreign substance, forces the immune system to kick into gear. Among regular, unstressed rats, the immune systems did just that, performing as they should have performed.

Real-world stress causes similar results. When a timid, insecure male rat is put in a cage with two dominant, turf-controlling rats, as in a 1989 University of Colorado at Boulder study, the bullies don't exactly bring out the welcome wagon. They quickly assert their dominance. While the space-invading newcomer rarely is injured, he does adopt the trademark rodent defeat posture of rolling over and lying on his back. If the confrontation plays out shortly after the victim gets a shot of KLH, his immune system's antibodies respond almost exactly as though he were exposed to electrical shocks: Levels of both IgM and IgG are lower and remain lower up to a month after the stressful encounter.

Does Stress Cause This Mess?

So stress and stress hormones coincide with illness in that stressful situations depress the immune system. Can we make the next leap in logic and say directly that the long-term lingering presence of stress-related hormones actually makes us sick? We believe so.

For a little evidence, let's visit your hometown sports team's locker room, where one of the body's three major stress hormones is a major presence. No, not because of the tension and anxiety associated with the big game but because of all of the injuries suffered in previous games. Athletes often take shots of cortisone, a compound closely related to the stress hormone cortisol, just before playing, to reduce inflammatory pain. Inflammation is, in part, a sign of an immune system at work.

Now let's leave the locker room and go across town to the recovery ward in a city hospital. Organ transplant patients there could well be getting injections of cortisol or a related compound to curb the body's innate desire to reject the foreign organ. That's how well-known the substance's immune-suppressing power is. Cortisol and other glucocorticoids deter both the creation and release of the immune system's major players, the cytokines. The fewer the cytokines, the less active the immune response.

The proposition is readily verifiable, demonstrated simply by administering drugs that block cortisol or other stress hormones, then creating a stressful situation and seeing what transpires. It's a pretty straightforward test: If the immune system still falters, then the blocked hormone probably isn't involved; if the immune system continues to work as well as it did before the stress, then the hormone probably is a culprit.

Evidence is back at the University of Colorado at Boulder. In 1995, a study was conducted in which rats were stressed with electric shocks and given the immune-stimulating drug KLH. Some of the rats then got a shot of a drug that prevented their bodies' ability to use the rodent equivalent of cortisol. Among those that received the cortisol blocker, their immune systems behaved perfectly, as if the rats weren't stressed at all. Those that didn't get the drug showed the typical signs of immune weakening. Many similar studies have demonstrated the same effect, also with the other two major stress hormones, epinephrine and norepinephrine. Inhibit their release, and the immune system will not stumble when you are stressed out.

Short-Term Benefits, Long-Term Hazards

In and of themselves, none of the reactions to stress are necessarily bad—in a momentary crisis. But what if they're prolonged and unresolved? What if your body does not get rid of the chemicals that make up the stress response? What if you can't make love no matter how sexy your partner looks? What if your cardiovascular system is agitated repeatedly for weeks and weeks without any resolution of the cause and return to normalcy? What if your immune system gets shortchanged, even slightly, for months?

If maintained for too long, the overall impact of stress is quite harmful indeed.

High blood pressure and heart disease. High blood pressure (hypertension) is the most significant risk factor for heart disease and stroke. A brief blood pressure elevation will pump more blood through your system and help you survive a physical threat. Assuming that it soon returns to normal, you'll probably suffer no long-term damage. But replace a quick battle against a saber-toothed tiger with a drawn-out, messy divorce that's accompanied by heated accusations, long-simmering acrimony, high-priced lawyers, and crying, confused children, and your tension level and blood pressure will be in the stratosphere for months, not minutes. The increased pressure could force a blood vessel to burst. If the ruptured vessel feeds your heart, you will have a coronary; if the vessel feeds the brain, you will have a stroke.

How Stressed Are You?

You no doubt know when you're stressed, but you can obtain a more objective measurement of how much tension you're experiencing and how much it's costing your immune system and health. After years of analyzing what changes are most stressful to people and what various disorders are likely to arise as a result, two researchers at the University of Washington School of Medicine in Seattle, Thomas Holmes, M.D., and Richard H. Rahe, M.D., devised what has become the standard professional gauge of stress and the likelihood that it will increase your risk of illness. The scale, originally published in 1967, was updated in 1997 by Dr. Rahe and Mark A. Miller, Ph.D., to account for the increase in stressfulness of life-changing events, and to be more specific about these events.

The simple assumption behind the Rahe Life Stress Scale is that change—any change—is stressful and, to at least some extent, likely to have an impact on health. Death of a child tops the list, followed by death of a spouse, death of a close family member, divorce, and separation. Interestingly, positive events are not necessarily stress-free. Getting married, getting pregnant, relocating to a new home, and even taking a vacation appear to be significant tension generators.

Though it's best to have your score interpreted by a psychologist or physician familiar with the scale, you can take the test yourself and obtain a rough estimate of how stressed you are. Check off each event that you've experienced over the past 12 months, add up the numbers, and consult the rating guide below. You may also find the scale on Dr. Rahe's Web site, www.hapi-health.com.

Interpreting Your Score

How many of these events have you experienced in the past year? Add up the numbers attached to each. This total is your Life Change Units (LCU). A score below 200 indicates that you have a low risk of a near-future illness. A score between 201 and 300 means that your odds of getting sick are moderate. A score between 301 and 450 points to elevated odds. Finally, if you score greater than 450, you are at high risk for imminent illness.

Death of a child 123	Moderately severe illness 44
Death of spouse 119	Birth of grandchild 43
Death of close family member .101	Loss/damage to personal
Divorce 96	property 43
Marital separation 79	Child leaves home 42
Jail term 75	Change in living conditions 42
Fired from work 74	Change in work responsibilities .41
Serious illness 74	Change in residence 40
Death of close friend 70	Personal relationship problems . .39
Pregnancy 67	Begin or end school 38
Birth or adoption 66	Trouble with in-laws or relatives . .38
Miscarriage or abortion 65	Major increase in income 38
Major business readjustment . . .60	Major purchase 37
Major loss of income 60	New close relationship 37
Parents divorce 59	Outstanding achievement 36
Relative moves in 59	Change in work conditions 35
Credit difficulties 56	Change in schools 35
Change in health or behavior of	Trouble at work 32
family member 55	Change in religious beliefs 29
Retirement 52	Change in church activities 27
Change to different line of work . .51	Change in personal habits 26
Major decision about future 51	Change in number of family
More arguments with spouse . . .50	get-togethers 25
Marriage 50	Change in political beliefs 24
Parent remarries 50	Vacation 24
Accident 48	Minor purchase 20
Partner begins or ends work . . .46	Less serious illness 20
Engagement 45	Minor violations of the law 20
Sexual difficulties 44	Taking courses 18

We all know someone taking medication to lower high blood pressure precisely to avoid these possibilities. The most commonly prescribed hypertension drugs are beta-blockers. They prevent two fundamental stress hormones, epinephrine and norepinephrine, from constricting blood vessels, speeding up heart rate, and otherwise affecting your body. (You're probably more familiar with epinephrine under its other name, adrenaline. Likewise, norepinephrine also is known as noradrenaline.) In this light, beta-blockers are essentially antistress drugs.

Atherosclerosis. Continued high blood pressure also causes minuscule rips and tears along the interior walls of the arteries. These chinks are ready-made nooks and crannies for cholesterol to lodge in, building up into blood-damming, artery-clogging plaque. Cholesterol, of course, is blood-borne fat, the level of which the stress response elevates as well (even independently of diet). If this process were not insidious enough, consider the very nature of stress hormones: They tend to assist in the production of the type of cholesterol that most likely clings to artery walls (low density lipoprotein, or LDL) and encourage the destruction of artery-cleansing, high-density lipoprotein, or HDL.

Diabetes. How about that rise in blood sugar? Not a problem— in a brief emergency. If you fight or flee, the physical activity will burn off surplus glucose, and everything should be fine. But if you sit and stew in your office cubicle for months on end and don't burn off the extra sugar in your bloodstream, you're essentially developing the primary symptom of diabetes, the fourth leading cause of death in the United States. A stress-filled life, especially if combined with a poor diet and a lack of exercise, is one of the bona-fide risk factors for this disease.

Brain damage, memory loss, and stroke. Surely the heightened senses and cognition that you feel when under the gun could not be bad in the long haul, right? Well, it is a gift horse in disguise, too. The effect comes courtesy of the stress hormone cortisol. Over time, cortisol apparently kills brain cells, according to research by Robert Sapolsky, Ph.D., a Stanford University biologist who has extensively studied the physiological consequences of stress. Cells that appear particularly vulnerable are located in the brain's hippocampus, an area critical for the formation of memories and one of the parts of the brain that deteriorates in Alzheimer's disease and other memory disorders. The implication is that chronic stress could be a contributing factor in Alzheimer's and other cognitive illnesses.

As mentioned, the greater flow of blood to your head increases pressure inside cranial vessels, leading to a greater risk that one might burst and cause a stroke. The brain is not unaware of the problem, and thus it reacts. Upon sensing the presence of elevated blood pressure, the brain releases chemicals that thicken and strengthen the walls of its vessels to guard against a potential rupture. In some instances, the thicker blood vessels press and impinge on nearby nerves, causing at least a headache. In other instances, the thickening results in a loss of blood vessel flexibility and elasticity, meaning they cannot adjust readily to surges of blood, which only magnifies the possibility that one could break open. Again, a defensive response backfires amid prolonged, unresolved stress, actually contributing to and magnifying the possibility of a stroke.

The Chronic Cost

Medicine generally recognizes that chronic stress is bad for health, but it has yet to grasp the full extent and all of the ramifications. High blood pressure is one thing, but the death of brain cells is quite another. Some of the documented changes induced by chronic stress are more severe and larger in both magnitude and duration than science originally thought, making stress reduction and the pursuit of pleasure far more important to your good health than is immediately apparent.

Hans Selye, M.D., the scientist who originally identified stress as a health threat, initially perceived it as an external threat that had to be fought off by the body through the secretion of hormones and other stress-related chemicals. He further proposed that prolonged tension simply exhausted the body's ability to secrete such substances. As Dr. Sapolsky and others have since demonstrated, this is not correct. You do not run out of stress hormones. Your body possesses the capacity to manufacture them as long as you are under duress.

Plain and simple, this fact is what makes a well-conceived short-term survival mechanism such a long-term threat. Physiologically, psychologically, and immunologically, your body, in a sense, is turning against itself. Exquisitely evolved self-defense measures ultimately prove to be self-destructive in the 21st-century world (they didn't help us much in the 20th century, either). This is why you must deliberately and consciously seek to counteract stress with pleasure.

Getting Connected . . .
with Less Stress

Stress is the antithesis of pleasure, not only definitionally but physiologically. Because of the opposing nature of the two parts of our autonomic nervous system, as discussed in chapter 1, stress and pleasure cannot coexist in the mind and body. So while stress inhibits your ability to have fun, pleasurable activities will reduce stress and the terrible toll that it takes on your immune system and your health.

Precisely what should you do? For one, read the rest of this book. All of its components are specifically designed to counteract stress and/or bulk up immunity. That's the principal and obvious recommendation, but for right now, we have a few other suggestions.

Recognize it. Listen to your body and learn to realize when you are under increased tension. The next time you've had a horrible day at work or a nasty fight with your mate, drive over to the neighborhood pharmacy or supermarket and stick your arm in one of those do-it-yourself blood pressure machines. Chances are you'll see a hypertensive spike.

For other measurements, you could tell your doctor that you want a test for the concentration of cortisol, a prime stress hormone, in either your blood or saliva. It's wise to first get a baseline cortisol measurement when you're generally not under any major undue tension. That way, as crises emerge in the future, you can get later tests to gauge the impact on your nerves and your immunity. For instance, with a basic reading of your cortisol level during relatively good times, you can see the expected cortisol spike if you later lapse into a deep funk, get fired, or lose your spouse.

Act on it. Don't make any excuses for why you can't have some fun. Don't say that you're too upset. Don't say that you just don't feel like it. Remember, behavior actually can change attitude.

Let the fun add up. As with the cumulative toll of stress, pleasure's effects on your mind and body are additive. Every little bit of fun and enjoyment adds up to a decreased strain on your immune system. So watch a funny movie. Go to a party. Meet up with friends at a bar. Dangle a string above your cat's head or throw a ball across the room for your dog to fetch. Cuddle up on the couch with your mate. Put on a favorite CD. Sit quietly and meditate. Have a glass of wine or a bottle of beer. Call your mother. Reorganize your coin collection. Take a long walk. Jog around the block a couple of times or go to the gym for a workout. Exercise is, in fact, a great stress reducer. It gets blood pumping in a more beneficial fashion, burns off those stress chemicals, and gives you a physical outlet for you to figuratively fight off or flee from your den of saber-toothed tigers.

Chapter 4

Music Soothes the Savage Breast

BUT CAN IT CURE THE COMMON COLD?

Music is the shorthand of emotion.
—Count Leo Nikolayevich Tolstoy, Russian novelist, philosopher, and mystic

The use of music in a healing capacity dates all the way back to biblical times, when David, lacking access to Prozac, played his harp to alleviate King Saul's depression. Ancient temples all over China, India, Egypt, and Greece were equipped with instruments intended to heal with music. It was no accident that Apollo was the God of both music and medicine, and that Aesclepius (arguably the world's first physician) employed music as a major curative tool. In 12th-century Europe, Abbess Hildegard von Bingen, perhaps the first music therapist, used melody to treat malady.

Soon after the middle of the 2nd millennium, however, physicians began to look askance at music as medicine. Not until the middle of the 20th century or so did music therapy reemerge as a legitimate field of study. Since then, science has documented music's ability to lift low spirits and reduce the secretion of chemicals associated with stress.

Listening to either classical music or classic rock improves exam scores among university students. Music sharpens attention, memory, and spatial ability. Listening to soft background music lowers blood pressure, pulse, and respiration among patients in the preop ward of a hospital. Classical music, one study concluded, increases a physician's surgical accuracy and speed. Everyone's job performance, in fact, improves if they whistle while they work. Music lulls the body into secreting feel-good, pleasure-promoting opioid peptides, thus elevating mood and helping deaden pain. The rhythm and syncopation help improve gait in people recovering from strokes and aid in steadying motor control among people with Parkinson's disease. Even children with autism benefit.

So while the concept is nothing new, the orchestral explosion in scientific research certainly is. "Take two tunes and call me in the morning" is not a bad prescription at all.

The Science behind the Music

Evidence of certain health benefits derived from listening to music is one thing; the notion that a melody might manipulate specific biochemicals in the body, such as immunoglobulin A (IgA), is quite another. It is still a somewhat odd idea today, let alone in 1988, when the idea emerged. Ours was the first-ever rigorously conducted, by-the-book scientific investigation into music's impact on immune health.

The primary obstacle in the investigation was twofold: We needed to rule out any particular feelings that might be evoked upon hearing a familiar tune or certain emotionally charged lyrics, and we needed to isolate music as the single, sole variable in any immune system shift.

The first part was easy: a song without words. If we were to play music with love-laden lyrics, Janice, who just met the love of her life, could very well swoon and swell with an excellent immune response, while Charlie, who just got dumped by his fiancée, could be expected to fall into a depressive funk.

The next part was more difficult. Sure, there are instrumental pieces in virtually every musical genre—pop, rock, country, blues, classical, disco, rap, and new wave. But how do you account for personal taste and emotional baggage here? If we put on, say, a Rachmaninoff recording or another classical piece, one listener may lapse into a blissful, immune-boosting state, while another, who hates classical music, may get bored, listless, or even irritated.

A conditioned response could also rear its ugly head here, too. If Eric, for example, heard the instrumental rendition on the radio frequently during the summer in which he fell madly in love with the woman who became his wife, we might never be able to wipe the immune-elevating smile off his face. But perhaps Linda, another study participant, may start to cry, for during that same summer her favorite uncle died after a long, debilitating illness.

Composing an Experiment

It would seem, then, that we had a real problem. No music, apparently, would meet our rigid criteria (the music should not evoke specific feelings, and it should be the only variable in the study), unless, of course, we composed our own.

And so we did. We decided to collaborate with a music theoretician. What we wanted, we explained, was a melody, not a series of sonatas with multiple movements, just a pure harmonic progression of notes repeated over and over for 30 minutes. Our colleague came up with a half-hour instrumental piece, performed beautifully on a Steinway, that no one had ever heard before, with four-part harmonization of ascending and descending notes, based on the choral melodies of

Bach and played in the very basic key of C major. He selected a Bach-like style for a specific reason. Among musical styles, it is familiar to a greater number of people, regardless of culture or educational background, than any other style in the history of the modern world.

So we were set—or were we? All we needed were two groups of people: one to listen to our new *Billboard* chart buster, and another to sit in silence for 30 minutes. But the thought occurred to us that perhaps anything to which we exposed our aural audience might influence immune parameters in some way. We decided to add a third group of study participants and alter just one variable: the tune's key, or, to be more technically correct, its mode. People in this group heard the exact same progression, except in the key of C *minor*.

Why C minor? Well, songs played in major keys typically sound bright and bold. Songs played in minor keys, in contrast, sound doleful and sad. Perhaps we could induce a bit of an immune decline with a sad-sounding song.

Good Vibrations

We were finally set. We had 25 people who would listen to the piano solo, 29 people who would listen to its minor-key equivalent, and 23 people who would sit comfortably in silence for 30 minutes. Before the immuno-concerto, we asked everyone to contribute a saliva sample to get a baseline measure of IgA. We played the 30-minute concert of sound or silence, and immediately after, we took separate saliva samples.

In examining the results, we discovered that those who savored the sounds of silence showed no changes in immune measurements. Nor did those exposed to our etude in C minor. However, those who listened to our collegiate classic in C major showed a significant jump in IgA measurements.

It was no fluke. What we found, according to statistical analyses, was that even if we performed this study 10,000 more times with 10,000 different groups of people, we'd likely get similar results. That's how significant the findings were. Nevertheless, we decided to conduct the experiment all over again, with a different group of people just to make sure.

The second time, true to the statistical analyses, we recorded the exact same results: Listening to the harmonic progression in C major increased IgA levels significantly. Mere exposure to resonant vibrations in the air influences one of the most important chemicals in the immune system. Imagine the incredible, widespread ramifications. But our excitement was tempered by dozens of questions that the results naturally raised: How long does the immune boost last? Would other forms of music accomplish the same thing? In particular, would music that we typically listen to on the radio or on CDs have a similar effect? And just what is it about our psychophysiological being that enables an interplay between our internal defense systems and these external "good vibrations"?

One day some 8 years later, we were contacted by someone from Muzak who caught wind of our work. The company, the premier purveyor of so-called elevator music, found our research of considerable interest and believed that some of its compositions might generate similar internal benefits on health. Would we, he asked, put some of Muzak's renditions of familiar songs to the IgA test?

Our immediate gut reaction was an emphatic "No!" Imagine the notion that elevator music might exert some sway on the majestic internal workings of the system that we had come to revere so. This was not acceptable. Bach was a worthy partner in this lofty scientific endeavor. But Muzak?

But while musing over the proposition, aesthetic tastes and cultural standards gave way to our scientific curiosity. We told the Muzak representative to send us a 30-minute tape of "music" that he thought might benefit the immune system. We soon received a half-hour cassette of what could best be characterized as smooth jazz. It was, though, definitely recognizable as Muzak, and it included instrumental versions of the Eagles song "Peaceful Easy Feeling" and Marvin Gaye's "What's Going On?"

In order to keep ourselves on safe, scientific ground, we wanted to double up on the control groups. Yes, we'd include a group of people who sat in a silent room. But we also wanted some folks to listen to a half-hour of other, non-Muzak smooth jazz taped off the radio. Moreover, to account for the possibility that perhaps ANY auditory stimulus might influence immune chemicals, we chose to include still another group of people who listened to an innocuous series of alternating hums and clicks. As before, everyone deposited saliva into a cup before and after the performance to get an IgA measurement. Here's what we documented.

- ◆ In the hum-click group, IgA fell by an average of 19.7 percent.
- ◆ Those who sat in silence experienced virtually no change in IgA.
- ◆ The people who heard the radio tape displayed a 7.2 percent average increase in IgA.
- ◆ Among the Muzak listeners, IgA jumped by an average of 14.1 percent.

As we learned previously, silence does not help your health. That much is clear. It won't hurt, but it won't help. Listening to discordant, nonmelodic noise apparently may unnerve you enough to weaken immune activity. Listening to songs on a smooth-jazz radio station seems to nudge immune parameters up a bit. But the Muzak doubled the immunity-improving impact of the commercial music and produced a statistically significant effect.

A Musical Boost?

While the results of our Muzak experiment were consistent with those of our initial experiment, they still didn't answer most of our questions. Louis Armstrong and John Coltrane can thus join our Bach-like tones in bolstering immunity, but who else might play in this all-star jam? Could Led Zeppelin sit in? How about L. L. Cool J and Neil Young? Is there room on stage for Kenny Rogers and Madonna? What about Frank Sinatra? What's more, is it all worth the effort? Just how long does the health promotion last? Until the song is over? An hour? A day? Should we give ourselves regular booster shots of music? And what truly orchestrates the immune performance? Is stress reduction or mood elevation wielding the baton, or is a more direct physiological process at work? As we prepared for our third experiment in 1997, we placed our bets on mood elevation and stress reduction.

As it turns out, we were wrong. Music didn't lower stress or make listeners any happier, because none of the participants described themselves as stressed or unhappy to begin with. The music did, though, elevate listeners' IgA readings dramatically.

We played some easy-listening contemporary soft rock produced by Muzak, including selections by Amy Grant, Lyle Lovett, Sting, and Alanis Morissette, for our audience, matched this time by just one group in the sound-free room. As before, everyone provided saliva samples immediately before and after the session, but we required everyone to return an hour later and again 3 hours later to give additional samples. On top of that, at each visit, we also asked everyone to gauge on a 10-point scale how happy or sad they were and how stressed or relaxed they felt. As it turned out, no one, neither before the test nor 3 hours later, was any more or less downhearted. Nor was anyone less tense before or after. Coming in and going out, these were all relatively happy, relaxed people.

That fact makes the results all the more amazing and intriguing because we could therefore attribute any marked shift in saliva measurements of IgA pretty reliably to what the study participants were (or were not) hearing. The study participants who listened to nothing displayed no noteworthy change in immune parameters immediately after the initial half-hour. That's not too surprising, given our earlier research. Among the soft-rock listeners, though, IgA

From Ear to Immunity

How can vibrating air molecules—which at its most basic are all that sound and song are—regulate the secretion of biochemicals? This field of investigation still is too new for definitive explanations. Yet science has some preliminary educated guesses.

Some have theorized that every one of our cells responds, positively or negatively, to different resonant tones. After all, the body does attune itself to certain rhythms. Heartbeat and respiration, for example, tend to synchronize themselves to the beat of whatever we happen to be listening to. It's also true that listening to some tunes makes us happy and content, which in turn triggers the body's release of feel-good opioid peptides.

What we know for sure is that sound triggers and influences certain neural projections throughout the brain. It only makes sense that these areas are sensitive to song, too. In fact, the same part of the brain (the right cerebral hemisphere) that music stimulates is the same part that's largely responsible for governing the slowdown of the immune system. Somehow, music may provide a buffer against the immune deceleration.

jumped by 27 percent. The elevation, although twice that recorded in the previous experiment, had come to be expected. What really astonished us were the immune changes documented in the following 3 hours.

An hour later, the music listeners' IgA readings had returned to normal, basically the same as before turning on the tape machine. Three hours later, the measurements remained unchanged. Now for the follow-up on the people who sat in silence for 30 minutes. An hour later, their IgA levels fell below the measurements recorded before the beginning of the experiment. Three hours later, the same measurements plummeted even lower. Given that all of the participants were assigned randomly to one of the two groups, the likelihood that these people all did something different from the other group in the intervening 3 hours to drive down their IgA levels borders on statistical impossibility.

The Meaning behind the Music

We have several fascinating results to account for; let's tackle them individually.

The big boost. In elevating a basic immune parameter, is soft rock more healthful than smooth jazz? Doubtful. We think that the difference reflects the pleasure of preference. Study participants may find soft rock more enjoyable to hear than smooth jazz. Other forms of music may have a positive influence but perhaps not to the same degree as if you listen to something that you like.

The inoculation effect. Note that IgA levels of both groups of participants dropped within an hour after the experiment. Whatever they were doing during those 60 minutes, it drove down their IgA. The difference was that the listeners' measurements returned to baseline, or normal, while those of the nonlisteners fell far below the norm. Three hours later, the people in the silent set continued to experience an IgA decline, and the others maintained their preexperiment levels. Music may not have elevated the immune chemical for very long, but every little bit helps, and it certainly seems as though it may have inoculated listeners from an inevitable decline later in the day. It sounds as though we may need a booster shot of Basie perhaps every hour or so to keep our natural disease-fighting defenses working optimally.

The stress connection. The people in our study were not tense or high-strung—they were students, after all—so it does not seem likely that the stress-reducing, mood-brightening qualities of music played a role in elevating IgA. It simply was not a factor in this study. This is not to say that music cannot tame tension and improve immune performance. In fact, that was the whole point of our next study.

The Power of Preferences

When we talk about preferences, we're talking about what you like, what pleases you, or what your pleasure is. This individualized component is so important because this is what is at the heart of most preferences. And preferences are paramount regarding much of what we find healthy for our immune systems. Certainly, when we talk about music being the influential immune system variable, we think that this is particularly true. While we don't have direct evidence here, a number of studies document the importance of musical preference as a variable influencing such positive states as relaxation and mood elevation.

So this may be a good place to take a closer look at preferences. Preferences are innate, acquired, and contextually or situationally determined. Our innate preferences tend to be more closely tied to our survival needs. We will function best in, and hence prefer, an oxygen-rich atmosphere. And so we will bring our own at altitudes where it thins out. We will eat objects that we can digest and absorb nutrients from. So when we're hungry, we prefer a cheeseburger to a rock. When we're thirsty, we prefer liquid to a cheeseburger, and when sexually aroused, we probably prefer a member of the opposite sex. These preferences are all geared toward the survival of the individual and/or the species, so they tend to have stronger innate components. But even here we must note that it's not all a genetic fait accompli. All people don't prefer the opposite sex, and nuances of preference for satisfying the need for food and water are innumerable, ranging from water to wine and berries to beef bourguignon. So actually, the majority of personal preferences are acquired, but some of these have very subtle and purposive innate, early developmental, and biological influences.

Let us look at food preferences. Early on in life, there is an innate preference for sweet tastes. Why? Probably because we don't want Junior to spit out sweet-tasting colostrum (mother's milk), which provides nourishment and pumps IgA into our systems—both of which provide survival value. But why does this sweet taste persist in many people? Maybe it's just due to early exposure or maybe it comes to be associated with Mom or the comfort of having one's needs met. Obviously, association is critical in the acquisition of preferences.

How about physical interpersonal attraction? Are there innately determined components? Probably. Facial symmetry is one variable positively correlated with attraction. It is predictive of better health and genes. An approximate 12-inch difference in hip-to-waist ratio in women is positively correlated with attractiveness. This is also positively correlated with good childbearing—survival of the species. And in chapter 5 you'll find information suggesting the possibility of individuals with complementary immune systems being attracted to each other—offspring survival advantage.

Other weird biologically based reasons for preferences exist. We talk about early separation of monkeys from their mothers in chapter 5. This brings a strong preference for alcohol later in life as self-medication for stress.

Let's take a closer look at variables that influence musical preferences. Early on, there's a preference for higher-pitched voices. This of course would be Mom. And since preferences frequently put smiles on our faces, this rewards Mom's attention to us and hence makes it more probable. This has survival value. Then again, consider the notion that most music that we listen to contains 70 to 80 beats per minute. Is this an accident, or is it because this encompasses the range of typical heart rate? And what about music at 60 beats per minute being relaxing and music at 90 beats per minute stimulating (60 beats is a slow heart rate; 90 beats is fast). And what about the notion of entrainment, where physical vibrations in the air affect things, including bodily systems, in ways that bring them into synchrony. Is all this just coincidence, or does it affect our musical preferences? We think that it's probably critical. Studies show that we have an affinity for heartbeat when we're born. We will even seek out Mom's left breast when nursing because it provides the sensation produced by the beat of her heart.

So, in part, our musical preferences probably have biological roots, but of course the opportunity for association and Pavlovian conditioning are enormously potent determinants, not to mention situation-specific preferences. Would most people enjoy the Requiem Mass music at a wedding or "Stayin' Alive" at a funeral?

Obviously, the combination of innate acquired and situationally determined preferences makes each individual enormously complex in this regard. Musical preference is no exception, but it appears to be a critical variable for determining effects on the immune system. Luckily, music seems to be preferred to silence or disharmonic sound for boosting the immune system in general.

Whistling (and Listening) while You Work

What would happen to immune fortification if a bunch of wired, stressed-out people listened to music? How might IgA levels change over time, among different age groups, and in a real-world situation? In 1997 and 1998 we got a chance to find out in a rather nerve-racking environment: a noisy, harried, hurried, frenzied nonstop newspaper office under the gun of a pending deadline. By any definition, this was a stress-filled, pressure-cooker environment. Ten news writers, five men and five women ranging in age from 23 to 38, volunteered for our study. Before turning on the smooth-jazz tape previously used, we took from everyone two different saliva samples a half-hour apart just to see how IgA might change naturally within a given period, then asked each journalist to rate his or her stress levels. We pressed the PLAY button, and when the tape was over, we twice gathered saliva samples, again 30 minutes apart, and asked the reporters to assess their stress.

What happened to the nerve-jarred journalists? We documented two rather impressive results. First, stress levels did not change in the half-hour before the music began. By the time the tape finished, though, the average tension level decreased substantially and persisted for the ensuing 30 minutes. Second, IgA levels dipped slightly in the time before the smooth jazzy sounds wafted their way through the newsroom but had increased markedly after the music ended and continued its ascent 30 minutes later.

By all rights, with the deadline looming, stress levels should have shot up, and IgA should have taken a plunge, if not while the tape played then certainly once it stopped. Instead, the exact opposite occurred, and the only factor likely to have enabled it was the music. It produced a sustained reduction in stress and a sustained increase in a basic element of immune health.

Why would IgA continue its climb in the newsroom but not among participants in our earlier study? We're not sure. It might have been the musical style (soft rock versus smooth jazz), age differences, the surroundings (real world versus a clinical setting), or the interaction with stress (or its absence). We speculate that the prolonged rise is related to the lingering influence of stress reduction.

Marching to the Beat of Your Own Drum

We broke ground in studying how music influences immune system components. In the years since our initial study in 1988, only a handful of other researchers have bothered to join the band, usually tying tunes to some other stress-reduction technique, such as relaxation, imagery, or mood manipulation. What they have discovered is that music, at least in part, can sway the immune system's release of not only IgA but also lymphocytes, neutrophils, and interleukin-1.

Coming Out of the Shell

Children with autism, a condition that is being increasingly linked to a host of immune components, behave better and perform better at such spatial-oriented tasks as block-building if they first listen to music, according to some very preliminary results of our newest study with a small sample of participants.

In a series of sessions over the course of a few months in 2000, we supervised two autistic children—a 4-year-old boy and a 6-year-old girl—in duplicating various block-building designs. Sometimes we preceded the session with 10 minutes of silence; sometimes we started off with 10 minutes of soothing, relaxing music; and sometimes we played 10 minutes of Mozart's Sonata in D Major for Two Pianos.

Compared with how well they did after sitting in silence, the children's ability to recreate the block designs (a reflection of spatial skills) improved after listening to either of the two musical selections, with Mozart rising to the top as the better performance enhancer. In addition, playing music corresponded to fewer incidences of inappropriate behavior among children with autism, including flapping their hands and aggressive actions (which are typical for some children with autism).

A groundswell of evidence links autism to the immune system as one possible causal factor in a number of ways, including deficiencies of certain immune components and the possible presence of immune-evading microorganisms in the brain. As for our study of better block-building, science knows that the neural circuitry involved in spatial thinking occurs primarily in the right cerebral hemisphere—the same part of the brain that is stimulated when you listen to music and the same part responsible for slowing down immunity. Coincidence? Perhaps, but we don't think so. Music, more probably, is stimulating the right cerebral hemisphere, and in some ways perhaps is buffering against an immune system slowdown—an added bonus.

Other studies support an immune benefit indirectly by demonstrating an effect on emotional states known to weaken our natural defenses. For instance, a 1998 study of 194 people, culled from church groups in seven different cities across the country, concluded that mood-modulating Mozart soothes tension and that grunge-rocking Pearl Jam excites aggression. Divvying up study participants along age lines between adults and teenagers, researchers from the Institute of HeartMath in Boulder Creek, California, found that Mozart's Piano Concerto in D Minor and his *Six German Dances* lessened fatigue, sadness, and tension significantly—across all age groups. Listening to songs on Pearl Jam's *Vitalogy* album tended to increase fatigue, tension, and hostility—states that tend to depress immunity—again, in both teens and adults.

Research findings on the impact of other stimulating styles of music (anything approaching 90 beats per minute) are mixed. A 1976 investigation concluded that stimulating music increases worry and emotionality. Other studies found that listening to stimulating music can enhance mood and decrease apathy. This was the case with a 1998 British experiment conducted by Maudsley Hospital and the School of Nursing at Queen's Medical Center at the University of Nottingham that examined the effects of disco music, heavy rock music, heavy rap music, and what was described as hardcore house music on a group of college students.

We may not be particularly enamored of house music, rap, and disco, so we might not personally understand why this music would strengthen immune parameters. But we trust the results of the study. It is another testament to taste. If you like the music, it's going to make you feel better, and thus it is likely to make your immune system perform better.

While the limited research supports what we have already learned, no one as yet can explain how or why music makes immunity merrier (see "From Ear to Immunity" on page 90). For practical purposes, it doesn't really matter—music muscles up the body's internal defenses. So turn on the stereo, take those old records off the shelf, and give yourself some old-time rock-and-roll immunity.

Getting Connected . . .
with Music

"'Fools,' said I, 'you do not know. Silence like a cancer grows.'" So sang Simon and Garfunkel in "The Sounds of Silence." Silence won't kill you, of course, or instigate tumor growth, but it's neither as pleasurable nor, certainly, as immune-promoting as a good set of songs. Our lives are filled with dissonance. For stability and sanity, we need a continuous, rhythmic, almost haunting can't-get-it-out-of-your-head theme resonating through our bodies. Music is the answer.

Please, please me. What kind of music do you like? Music that appeals to you and pleases you. Perhaps it's a catchy, infectious riff or chorus. Perhaps it's the dulcet trills of tinkled piano keys. Maybe it's the romantic massage of violin strings or the searing, soaring sounds of an electric guitar. Maybe it's a primal, tribal drumbeat; a mournful, soulful trumpet; or a lonesome, emotional harmonica wail. Whatever it might be, something inside you is attracted to certain sounds and combinations of notes. It might make others grimace and cover their ears, but you like it and enjoy it. Musical preference is different in each of us. If it makes you happy, it may positively influence your immune system.

Turn on, tune in, change channels. Listen to what you like. It's fine to turn on your favorite radio station, but definitely tune to something else when a song comes on that you don't like. Selecting your own music allows you to control your environment, which in itself is beneficial to the immune system.

Pop on a platter. The radio is convenient, but it's better to build your own music collection. As opposed to just listening to the radio, playing your own records, CDs, and tapes may boost your immune parameters even higher. Why? Again, you especially like that music, and you control what you hear. In addition, it's uninterrupted by commercials and announcements.

You better shop around. Pick a day, perhaps a rainy Saturday or Sunday, and go to the mall or your favorite music store. Indulge yourself by buying a few favorite discs that you've always wanted to own. Acquiring things is, in and of itself, a great emotional lift. Don't kid yourself, guys: You love to shop too. It just depends on what you're shopping for.

Trade tunes. Book clubs are great. Tupperware parties are . . . well, they're okay, too. But regular music exchanges are excellent ways to expand your aural horizons. Trade CDs and tapes with your friends. Join internet discussion groups devoted to your favorite musicians. Develop e-mail friendships with like-minded souls who like to discuss particular artists and who like to trade sound files.

Wake up to your favorite song. Start your day with an immediate immune boost. Get a CD player with an alarm that allows you to program the first song you hear in the morning. Greet the day with your favorite feel-good music.

Don't rock around the clock. From tempo, pitch, timbre, and tone to sound, style, and melody, so many variables figure into your enjoyment of a song and its effect on you emotionally and thus immunologically at any particular time of day. Experiment with your own musical programming based on the time of day, your mood, and what you're doing. Don't, for example, listen to Chopin's nocturnes first thing in the morning. When you wake up, put on something energetic. Fuel your midday fires with still more energetic, enjoyable music. Sing along with favorite tunes if you're engaged in physical work, but stoke the flames with some classical music if you're mired in more intellectual endeavors. At the end of the day, start to mellow out with some Crosby, Stills, Nash, and Young; and put the Chopin nocturnes on in the hour before you go to bed.

Customize your concerts. Make recordings of your favorite music, using a cassette recorder, CD burner, MP3 player, or your home computer. One tape, CD, or program could consist entirely of relaxing music to help you unwind after one of those days; another could contain stimulating, cheerier tunes by which to exercise or clean the house. Let your own preferences guide you. All we would suggest is that music with 60 beats or less per minute tends to relax, while music of more than 90 beats per minute tends to rev you up.

Take in tunes before you toil. Listen to a favorite tape, CD, or radio station on your way to work. One study demonstrated that listening to enjoyable music primes your pump for a better on-the-job performance. It's the breakfast of immune champions, too.

Avoid fingernails on the chalkboard. If you work in a loud, noisy environment, ask your boss if you can listen to music with a set of headphones. If not, get a set of earplugs. Noise is nerve-jarring aural agitation.

Learn how to play. You don't have to become a Les Paul or Yehudi Menuhin. Whether it's the guitar or the violin, or for that matter a harmonica, the spoons, or a single string tied to a broom handle that's lashed to an old metal washtub, learn how to play a musical instrument. We've all got the music in us, and belting out a song can only do you good.

Name that tune. Play music associated with positive, happy events in your life. Don't listen to the song that was on the jukebox when the love of your life broke up with you.

Hear the hidden message. No, we're not talking about playing records backward to hear satanic commands or clues about Paul Mc-Cartney. We're talking about deliberately conditioning yourself to associate certain songs with certain emotional states. Put on one of your very favorite mellower songs, then immediately sit down or lie down, close your eyes, and instill a deep state of relaxation. Breathe deeply and slowly, relax your muscles progressively, meditate, whatever you choose. Do this repeatedly, a dozen times or more. Eventually, you'll learn to associate this song with calmness and relaxation. Every time you hear the song, even when you don't lie down on the sofa, you'll tend to settle down and soothe your rattled nerves automatically. Once your mind learns the association, you can take advantage of this conditioning whenever you need it: right before an important sales presentation, just before you ask that special person for a date, on the way to a job interview—whenever you need to counteract stress.

Move to the music. Tap your toes. Stomp your foot. Drum your fingers on the steering wheel. Nod your head in sync with the beat. Dance in the streets. Movement helps counteract depression. The exercise is good, a release for your stress-tightened muscles. If you have a mate, put on "When a Man Loves a Woman" and snuggle up. Pick a Saturday night and orchestrate a dinner-dance. Invite a few couples over, eat a sumptuous meal, then roll up the rug and roll out the music. If you don't have a partner, don't worry. Put on "Disco Inferno" or "Xanadu" and dance, dance, dance.

Sing along. As with dancing, crooning along with a song involves you more emotionally with the music and allows you to exercise more muscle (both vocal and immune). This is speculative, but we think that the combination of music and "letting it out" may be a particularly potent combination for immune health. So sing in the shower. Sing in the rain, if you like. The latter would be a nice homage to Gene Kelly.

Chapter 5

The Pleasure of Touch

LOVE, SEX, AND SOCIAL SUPPORT

*One must not lose desires. They are mighty stimulants
to creativeness, to love, and to long life.*
—Alexander A. Bogomoletz, Ukrainian scientist and academician

Do you have a lover? Does he or she prop you up emotionally?
Is your partner warm and affectionate? How is life in the bedroom? Are you divorced? Were you close to your parents? How many friends do you have, and how often do you see them? Can you turn to them and confide in them when life gets rough?

What does your sex life have to do with the camaraderie of a coffee klatch? They differ in degree and form, but they're both expressions of love and emotional support.

Lovers, friends and family definitely can drive us to distraction at times, but we need them. We function best and are happiest and healthiest when we have people in our lives. Sure, we need solo time too, but chronic loneliness, experienced by millions, can actually be a health risk, associated with higher instances of illness and a greater likelihood of death. Loving and living in a social network of friends and family improves your health and your chances of recovering from illness. We can't always make a direct connection to better immune function, but the health rewards are dramatically clear.

Social Immunity: Health Security

Apologies in advance to Carole King and James Taylor for the paraphrasing, but when you're down, troubled, and need a helping hand, when nothing seems to be going right, do you have a friend? Better yet, friends? Do you have people to lean on, people to talk to you, people to tell you that, despite your doubts, everything will work out? That's emotional support, and it can come from anyone—a lover, parents, other family members, friends, neighbors, acquaintances at the gym or country club, members of a church group, coworkers, the bowling league, even seemingly impersonal cyberfriends on the internet.

The bigger your support network, the better your health, according to numerous scientific investigations. Social support elevates a variety of immune parameters and prolongs survival from the deadliest of afflictions, including heart disease, cancer, and AIDS. Medicine has had solid documentation of the value of social support at least since the 1960s, when Lisa Berkman, Ph.D., from the University of California, Berkeley, compared the health states of more than 7,000 men and women in Alameda County, California, with the extent of their social support. Whether from family, friends, or church, people with fewer interpersonal interactions were two to three times more likely to die within 9 years from cancer, heart disease, or a whole host of other maladies. In and of itself, that's rather strong evidence, but it becomes even more powerful upon closer inspection. The number of social ties was a more accurate statistical predictor of health than factors that you'd think were far more crucial: age, current medical status, alcohol consumption, and even smoking.

A long list of other studies offers similar findings. The sentiment may be a little schmaltzy these days, but Barbra Streisand was right: People who need (and seek out) people really are the luckiest people in the world—and the healthiest.

Disease and the Dorm Mouse

When it comes to support networks, we're basically no different from our counterparts in the animal world. Rodents need friends too. As an elegant series of studies demonstrated, mice fight cancer better when they interact in healthy ways with other mice. Researchers injected mice with a tumor-generating substance, then manipulated their living conditions. Some lived alone; others lived in the cozy atmosphere of group animal housing. Mice accustomed to fraternization invariably grew the largest tumors after being moved to their own individual—and lonely—dwellings. Mice that originally lived alone but later were relocated among their peers had the smallest tumors. Tumor growth fell somewhere in the middle for those rodents that always lived alone or always lived with others.

It is not just the presence of social interaction that improves health and deters cancer. It's the quality of the social interaction. As you might expect, living with others is one thing; living with others in stability and peace is quite another. Studies with mice show that living in a hostile, threatening environment actually promotes tumor growth, while living in harmony with your fellow mouse slows the cancer's spread. The same can and should be expected with your social relationships. If they're good, they can be very good for your health. If they're bad, they may adversely affect your health.

A Many-Splendored Thing

Poets spend careers writing about it. Musicians pen songs about it. How many songs or poems are dedicated to cars, politics, or hockey teams? A few, to be sure, but the vast majority are about looking for love, declaring love, missing your love, being wronged in love, and trying to choose between two loves. Without love songs, FM radio would be virtually silent. All of us strive to find love. Countless volumes have been written about the psychological and emotional aspects of love, but only recently have a few researchers begun to consider the physiological effects. Without question, something physical happens when we experience or express love. We get that warm, fuzzy feeling inside. The heart races, the eyes glisten, palms moisten with sweat, and that practiced debonair James Bond smoothness somehow translates into fumbling idiocy when we open our mouths. But what exactly occurs physiologically? And might it be good for your health?

Generally, yes. People in love tend to live longer and are healthier. But because this field of investigation is still in its infancy, science can't offer solid explanations for why. One reason for the dearth of data is that love is difficult to study. You can lock people in a room and expose them to music for 30 minutes, but you can't shove people in a room and tell them to "love" for the next half-hour. Another problem is definitional: What kind of love are we talking about—romantic love, parental and familial love, platonic love among good friends, or the altruistic love of caregivers and volunteers? And how do you know if someone is truly in love?

We could study married people or other couples involved in close romantic relationships. Presumably, they are in love. How, though, do you isolate love's impact on health? Marriage is intimately linked (or should be) with emotional support and sex. How do you separate those aspects from love? Sure, couples undoubtedly exist who do not offer one another emotional support and haven't engaged in sex for years. They probably don't love each other all that much, either. Sex can perhaps be factored out, but emotional support cannot. It's an intrinsic component of what we think of as love.

Overall, couples in good marriages or other intimate relationships are healthier than their unattached peers. They live longer. They have more natural killer-cell activity in their immune systems. Cancer doesn't progress as rapidly in their bodies. Good relationships buffer them against a variety of illnesses. Compared with unmarried people, those who have tied the knot also come through hospital stays more successfully. They generally have less serious diagnoses upon admission, stay in the hospital for less time, and are less likely to die while hospitalized. They're also less likely to be placed in nursing homes upon discharge.

Of course, two rings, a garter belt, and an expensive photo album won't guarantee better health. After the honeymoon really is over, couples must handle the everyday aspects of marriage. Just being married is not enough to boost your health. Research suggests that a bad marriage or chronic fighting is actually bad for the immune system.

Getting out of a bad relationship (and eventually into a good one) may be one of the best things you can do for your sanity and immunity. But it will not come quickly, and it does not come without cost, according to Ronald Glaser, Ph.D., and Janice Kiecolt-Glaser, Ph.D., researchers at Ohio State University in Columbus. In a series of experiments, the husband-and-wife team has documented a wide range of weaknesses in immune function among people going through divorces or separations, two of the most stressful episodes to experience. A return to normalcy, emotionally and immunologically, generally takes several years, and having a good social network for support helps cushion the blow.

Loss of Love . . . And Loss of Life
Charles Schulz succumbed to cancer the very night his final *Peanuts* comic strip rolled off the presses. A great love in his life

had "died." We've all heard similar stories of someone dying not long after a spouse or longtime companion dies. They just don't seem to want to live anymore. Their partner's death drained all the life out of them. And it's no coincidence. Though no direct causal connection can be made, the statistical evidence is solid—and amazing.

The probability of death skyrockets after a partner dies. In fact, it increases ninefold in the 12 months following the death, according to one estimate. That holds true despite age and health status. Grieving spouses, particularly men, suffer higher-than-expected rates of infectious diseases. Some 67 percent of all men, according to calculations from another study, experience a decline in health in the year following the deaths of their wives. The dip may not be significant if you're 35 years old and relatively healthy in the first place, but it could spell the difference between life and death if you're 65 or older and already in declining health.

Lab tests document the corresponding decline in immune power. The drop isn't so significant immediately after the loss of a loved one, probably because of the flurry of activity and the comfort of friends and family. All of that social support helps buffer the punishing blow to your immune system. Six to eight weeks afterward, though, the reality of the loss begins to sink in. That is when specific disturbances in just about any aspect of immunity can be measured, according to another group of experiments by Dr. Glaser and Dr. Kiecolt-Glaser.

What is the active factor? Is it the loss of love? Is it the loss of a reason for living? Is it the loss of your one-on-one social network? Is it the stress that comes with the upheaval in virtually every aspect of life? The figurative death of a relationship through divorce certainly is tension-generating, but the literal death of a partner or another close loved one is the most traumatically stressful event you can endure.

Moms, Dads, and Monkey Love

How did we first learn to love? From our parents, of course. Are we healthier if we learned to have close, loving relationships with our mothers and fathers? Apparently so. The correlation was easy enough to make for a quartet of Harvard University researchers. In the late 1980s they randomly selected 126 men who were Harvard students back in the early 1950s and asked them how warm and close their relationships were with their parents as they grew up. They then looked at the former students' current health. Of the men who did not enjoy very close relationships with their mothers and fathers, an astonishing 100 percent had been diagnosed with a serious disease. Those who had close relationships with one parent but not the other were a little better off; about 75 percent had a serious illness. Among the men who enjoyed great relationships with both parents, only 40 percent had major health problems. This is powerful stuff. How much love you and your parents share when you are young seemingly affects your health when you're older.

It also might influence your susceptibility to stress and your predisposition to addiction. Here we turn to a few animal experiments. Let's start with the notion that love may be as basic a physiological need as food. That was the unexpected conclusion of studies conducted back in the 1950s and 1960s by behavioral psychologist Harry Harlow, Ph.D., of the University of Wisconsin in Madison. As a behaviorist, he believed, like the American psychologist B. F. Skinner, that all behavior, including love, was the learned, acquired result of positive rewards and reinforcements and negative deterrents. Babies love their mothers, he proposed, because mothers provide food.

In a series of experiments, Dr. Harlow gave infant monkeys a choice between two artificial "mothers." One was soft and covered with cloth; the other was essentially a wire-mesh form. No matter which mother had the food, the baby monkeys spent all of their time clinging to the soft cloth. In fact, when the wire mother had the food, the infants would run over to it, grab a quick bite to eat, then immediately scurry back to the cuddly creature that it preferred to think of as Mom. To the researchers' surprise, the dependence on food is not the reason we come to love our mothers.

Apparently we have an innate need for comfort and love, and their absence could present dire consequences. That conclusion seems clear from experiments by two researchers from the National Institutes of Health. They separated 40 monkeys from their mothers immediately following birth, raising them for a month in a special monkey nursery. The infants then were raised in groups of three. Meanwhile, an additional 57 monkeys were raised and nurtured naturally by their mothers. After 6 months, the babies were exposed to the severe stress of a brief separation from either their mothers or their group peers. All of the animals displayed elevations in the stress hormone cortisol, but the chemical increased far more dramatically in those that never had mothers. Perhaps being raised without love, these findings suggest, renders us more susceptible to stress.

That tentative conclusion is borne out by subsequent studies 3 to 5 years later. The monkeys, now young adults, were put in a room in which they could voluntarily consume either water or alcohol. On average, the monkeys raised without mothers drank more alcohol than those that benefited from warm, caring parents. What's more, those that displayed the highest cortisol responses during the years-earlier separation experiment drank the most alcohol. In other words, their exaggerated stress response later predicted their alcohol consumption. Monkeys aren't people, of course, but the results ring true. It sounds quite plausible that people raised without maternal love may be more susceptible to stress and more likely to self-medicate by turning to alcohol or drugs.

Love, Immune-System Style

Love may certainly influence your immune system, even if science is not sure exactly how. Amazingly, the immune system, in return, may actually determine with whom you fall in love. You think it might be that killer body, those chiseled features, those gorgeous eyes, or that sparkling personality. In reality, it could be a great set of B cells, some prolific T cells, and immunoglobulin A (IgA).

In a 1997 study at the University of Bern in Switzerland, women were asked to smell various T-shirts that had been worn by men, then rate how pleasing they found the scents. Consistently, women said that they preferred the scent of shirts worn by men whose immune systems happened to be the most genetically different from theirs.

Why would this make sense? If you procreate with someone whose immune system differs from yours, your child will likely possess the immunity of both parents and be generally more healthy. On some instinctive, primitive level, the person we consider attractive and come to love is the person we think can best help us produce the healthiest kids. Now, in terms of romance, this isn't the stuff of an Air Supply song, and yet it may be true. Of everybody you've known, met, and dated, the one who ended up being the One has not only looks, brains, and personality, but the right phagocytes, too.

Selling Sex and Science

Sex saturates our airwaves, both visually and audibly. Exposed cleavage and well-muscled bodies are all over television. Billboards and magazine ads sport beautiful, sexy people who want you to buy the car that they drive, shop where they shop, and shampoo with the product that makes their hair gorgeous. Advertising and entertainment employ sex because it sells. It works. It strikes an ingrained,

Sex: A Fountain of Youth?

Research by neuropsychologist David Weeks, Ph.D., indicates that sex can make you look younger. In the book *Secrets of the Superyoung*, written with Jamie James, Dr. Weeks describes a 10-year survey that he conducted with 3,500 people from the United States, Great Britain, and the rest of Europe. Both men and women who reported having sex on average four times per week (twice as much as average), looked approximately 10 years younger than they really were, according to volunteer raters.

Dr. Weeks believes that hormones, such as growth hormone, released during sex are partially behind the effect. He cautions, however, that casual sex with multiple partners may be stressful and lead to premature aging. So get together with your partner, find some candles and music, and plan a romantic evening (or several!).

innate chord that nature installed eons ago to ensure the survival and propagation of our species.

Given something so fundamental to our very existence, why did research into human sexuality begin in earnest only in the last 100 years? Because it has always been, and probably always will be, something so intimate, so private and personal, that people just don't want to talk about it. John B. Watson, Ph.D., a highly influential American psychologist at the beginning of the 20th century, lost his job at Johns Hopkins University because he attempted to research the mechanics of the sexual response scientifically—with the help of his female grad student.

Serious, sober scientific investigations into sex really began in the 1940s, with groundbreaking studies by Alfred Kinsey, Ph.D., published in the 1950s, and continuing with additional pioneering work by William H. Masters, M.D., and Virginia Johnson. This pair documented that the gradual buildup and release of pleasure of the sexual response consists of four phases: excitement, plateau, orgasm, and resolution. All stages feature marked changes in the body, changes that affect the immune system. The intense physical pleasure and feeling of deep personal connection should be the first clues that sexual activity would influence immunity, but the physiological alterations offer more support: Heart rate and blood pressure increase dramatically, immune-bolstering endorphins are released, and orgasm reduces stress and tension. As with love, it's difficult to isolate any one factor as the key to the immune elevation. Is it purely one or more of the physiological changes? Is it merely the physical activity, the exercise, that tends to strengthen our natural defenses? We suspect that any health improvement derived from sex comes from a combination of the physiological changes and the feelings of love and interpersonal closeness.

Similarly, Candace Pert, Ph.D., in her book *Molecules of Emotion*, points out that in animal studies, levels of endorphins in the bloodstream skyrocket after orgasm. More evidence that sex does more than just make you feel good.

From a somewhat different angle, Barry Komisaruk, Ph.D., of Rutgers University in Newark, New Jersey, proposes that we need love and physical intimacy to prevent sickness. A psychologist and neuroscientist who has studied love, sex, and orgasm for a number of years, Dr. Komisaruk suggests that the entire physical and emotional experience of sex is necessary sensory stimulation that, if lacking, can pose problems. A neural mechanism may exist that causes psychosomatic illnesses if a person is deprived of love. In the absence of pleasurable sensations, the mind tries to generate some sort of sensory stimulation but ends up creating physical symptoms. In short, a lack of love in its many manifestations may make you sick.

Interested in the theory that lack of love can make you sick, and particularly intrigued by Dr. Dean Ornish's thoughts on the link between intimacy and health in his book *Love and Survival*, we sat down and planned an experiment of our own. We wanted to focus on intimate, romantic love and how it might sway our favorite indicator of immune health, IgA. We had 112 study participants, both men and women, fill out several questionnaires asking if they were in a long-term relationship, how long they've been in it, and how they felt about it. Then we asked them to rank their various levels of intimacy, passion, and commitment based on something called the Triangular Love Scale created by Robert Sternberg, Ph.D., of Yale University. We asked how many times they had intercourse during an average week and how satisfied they generally were with their sex lives.

We found several fascinating associations between the frequency of sex and immune strength. It was remarkable for two reasons: First, that a definite connection existed at all, and second, that it wasn't a simple more-is-better correlation. People who reported one or two sexual episodes per week enjoyed, among other things, higher IgA readings than those who engaged in no sexual contact or sexual contact less than once a week. They also had much higher measurements of this immune marker than those who had sex three or more times weekly. In fact, the people who were more sexually active had IgA levels comparable to those who were not sexually active. Plotted out graphically, the diagram would resemble an inverted U. The group in the middle had stronger IgA concentrations—about 30 percent more—than either of the two extremes. (Interestingly, the typical man—and presumably the typical woman—has sex an average of 1.5 times a week, according to a survey published in *Men's Health* magazine.)

Sexual Frequency: Solving the Riddle of the Middle

In analyzing our findings, we attribute the IgA improvement recorded in the once-or-twice-a-week middle group as opposed to those who did not have sex at all during an average week to the many positive effects of being in a relationship. The many psychological benefits presumably translate into physiological benefits. The phys-

Setting the Fire

If your sex life isn't as pleasurable as it used to be, take comfort in knowing that you are not alone. Take even more comfort (and pleasure!) in discovering that you can easily fan the flames of desire—and enhance immunity as a bonus—by remembering just a few simple tips.

Giving and receiving. Sometimes providing pleasure to a loved one can be as pleasurable as receiving it. When you're in a particularly giving mood, set a night aside specifically to provide pleasure to your partner. But make note of this and call in your markers on a night when you feel particularly interested in being on the receiving end, from your favorite meal to your favorite position. And you won't have to lift a finger; nothing but pleasure will be yours.

Looking good. Now and again, take time to make the perfect presentation to your partner—from hair to clothes to verbal communication to olfactory stimulation (smell) to body language—and derive great pleasure from the seductive delight that you elicit.

Variety. Enjoy nights or days when you don't plan anything the same in your encounter—from location to position. See how many different angles you can use to address the different opioid peptides, opioid peptide receptors, neurotransmitters, and neuromodulators of pleasure. Don't let your brain build up tolerance to the same stimulus conditions and hence diminish pleasure.

Spontaneity. Sometimes nothing excites pleasure molecules like a good old spontaneous appearance in the nude.

Foreplay. This is critical. Why? Because it heightens pleasure. And it's a good opportunity for synergy—giving and receiving, looking good, variety, and spontaneity all rolled into one.

ical act of sex itself also probably contributes to the IgA boost. Unfortunately, more bedroom activity does not translate into increased immunity function. For reasons we can only speculate about, more means less. It could simply be too much of a good thing bringing diminished returns. It could be fatigue or performance anxiety (too

Mother Teresa's T Cells

Did Mother Teresa have a more powerful immune system than the average person? She certainly lived to a ripe old age. We can't answer the question directly, because the literature on the health effects of spiritual, altruistic love is even more scarce than that on romantic and familial love. We do know, however, that *watching* Mother Teresa in action can elevate immune activity. In a study of people who viewed a film of Mother Teresa caring for the sick in Calcutta, their immunoglobulin A (IgA) levels rose significantly. No such changes were recorded when an audience watched a less loving movie.

tired from repeatedly trying to get it right). It could be some unknown other behaviors in which the thrice-weekly crowd engages.

Buried amid our piles of data, though, were some interesting relationships that show up only among people in the frequent-sex group (more than two times per week). Remember, we initially were examining love, and thus we had asked how much in love the study participants believed themselves to be and how secure they felt in their relationships. Well, among the frequent-sex group, the stronger they professed their love, the lower their IgA readings. The immune marker also was lower the more they claimed to be sexually satisfied by their relationships. Lots of sex, lots of professed love = lower IgA.

The conundrum made us wonder if these were anxious people engaging in sexual activity not out of actual love or attachment but rather out of insecurity. Perhaps there was anxiety and stress over the uncertainty of the relationship. Maybe they were having sex frequently as a cover-up and substitute for something else, such as communication or true affection. Similarly, couples in long-term, seemingly loving and romantic relationships who never have sex also, with certain exceptions, can be expected to have some sort of underlying, unaddressed issues.

Which brings us back to the healthier middle. Maybe it is not even the sex per se that contributes to their immune boost. Perhaps couples who have sex just once or twice a week are simply in healthier, more secure relationships and have nothing to prove. It may be their mutual love and contentment. We are not even certain that the immunological benefit applies to all people. Our study participants were all very much alike. All were college students no older than 23. Only one was married, and none described themselves as homosexual. We have yet to attempt testing our findings among older people, married couples, and homosexuals. Would our results hold true? Maybe, maybe not. If, for example, you're now 45, think back to a relationship you had in college. Other than the fact that you probably attend fewer keg parties these days, do you and your current mate have a similar relationship? The answer is almost certainly no, and the nature of that relationship may, for better or worse, influence sexual behavior's sway on your immune system.

Different Strokes?

We received a fair measure of publicity from this study and consented to doing a number of interviews. One of us was placed in a most uncomfortable position by a "Morning Zoo" disc jockey from a radio station in Florida. After asking about orgasm, the shock-jock then proceeded to berate his mate for his being sick all the time due to a "lack of action." Well, we walked ourselves right into a logistical minefield on this one, and now we have to confront a number of legitimate scientific questions for which, at this juncture, we frankly don't have the answers.

◆ Is it the entire sexual encounter, or is there something immunologically special about orgasm?

◆ Does the sex have to be intercourse? Will oral sex suffice? What about anal sex?

◆ If we've already had sex twice this week, should we take a cold shower when we're in the mood again?

◆ Does masturbation count? Or are love and physical contact critical?

◆ Moral and legal concerns notwithstanding, should a single, lonely person patronize prostitutes or engage in casual sex to help stay healthy? Or must the sex be with a loved one?

◆ Do immune-related differences exist between heterosexuals and homosexuals?

There probably is no magic number of times a week to have sex for optimum health and peak immune function. The number of weekly encounters reflects a thousand different variables for both partners. People in healthy relationships probably have sex a few times a week as a matter of course. We doubt that any huge differences in immunity potential are triggered by different kinds of sex. As for masturbation, there's probably an immune benefit from the pleasure and the release of tension, but the effect is likely to be somewhat less than with the warm, physical contact of a loving partner. And what of prostitution? In our humble scientific opinions, we'd guess that the guilt, shame, potential legal bills, and threat of a police record would outweigh any benefits of the sex.

Getting Connected . . .
with Touch

There's more than one way to put the touch on your immune system. Improving your sex life, seeking out more tactile pleasures, getting into shape, and expanding your social circle are just some of the possibilities that can raise your parasympathetic nervous system to new heights.

There's someone for everyone. That's what Mom always said, remember? If you're unattached and alone, never lose sight of the fact that you can and will meet that special person.

Get out there. A potential partner will not spontaneously enter your house uninvited. (These people are called burglars, and they unquestionably will not make good mates.) You have to go out, get involved, do things, and surround yourself with people who share your interests. Go to parties. Join a book discussion group. Yes, even place a personal ad. Once you screen out the Hannibal Lecters of the world, you may meet someone nice. We all know a single, lonely person who claims to be happy. We also know people who gripe about being alone and then, consciously or unconsciously, structure their lives to guarantee further loneliness and isolation.

Try to work it out. Bad relationships damage you psychologically, immunologically, and perhaps even physically. If there's a strain in your relationship with someone, try to work it out. Talk, communicate, open up, and share feelings. Try to reconcile differences. If that's difficult for either of you to do, consider going to a counselor.

Unburden yourself. Seek out emotional support from close friends and family members. Even if no solutions are identified, it still feels good to get matters off your chest. This recommendation goes double for guys. New research concludes that women seek out friends and social support when under stress far more easily than men. This could account for why women generally cope better with stress.

Break a tie that binds. If your relationship is horribly unsalvageable, if the love really has dissipated, you may need to consider a separation or divorce. The toll, emotionally and financially, could be quite draining, and it may not soon pass, but you'll position yourself ultimately to find a better, more loving, more compatible companion.

Become a volunteer. Because love and caring even on a much less personal basis seem to change immune strength positively, become a volunteer for a charity that helps people. You could teach people to read, participate in building houses for the poor, coach a youth sports team, or help out at a nursing home. Acts of caring and kindness are good for you and the object of your attention. And besides, you might meet a fellow Good Samaritan and strike up a romance.

Chapter 6

In Praise of Pets

YOUR IMMUNE SYSTEM'S BEST FRIEND

Animals are such agreeable friends—
they ask no questions, they pass no criticisms.
—George Eliot, *Mr. Gilfil's Love Story*

It was a beautiful fall evening in October as we sat in Carl's den discussing the vagaries of cytokine communication, the reinforcement schedules (reward rates) of casino slot machines, and what the Philadelphia Eagles need to do to win games. "Only two psychologists could take the fun out of a slot machine," Carl's wife noted.

Carl's dog, SuSu, trotted into the foyer and settled down on the ceramic tile. During a few minutes of lively conversation about interleukins and the West Coast offense, I noticed that SuSu had inched her way toward the den and finally placed her front paws on the edge of the carpeting that separates the den from the foyer. Seeing the advance peripherally, Carl gazed at her sternly while at the same time, with voiced raised, admonished her to "Get your paws off that carpet!" Without hesitation (actually, as if struck by lightning), SuSu jumped up and removed her paws from the carpet. She is not permitted in the den, but will, on occasion, test the waters, which always produces the same result.

People never cease to be amazed by SuSu's command of the English language. Of course, it was not the spoken word but Carl's facial expression and tone of his voice that motivated her response. In fact, Carl has demonstrated this fact on occasion by, in the same strict tone, substituting the words "Are you having a nice day?" for the command "Get your paws off the carpet." Whatever the words, SuSu responded the same: She retreated.

Lest you have conjured up an image of a mean man who is overly harsh with his pet, let's dispel that notion, for later that same evening SuSu lay comfortably in her master's lap as he stroked her lovingly. Did he love this dog, or had he simply read the research that suggested that exposure to a pet might have a positive influence on his blood pressure and heart rate? And, come to think of it, might it influence his immune system? The man and the dog had sustained, entertained, and nurtured each other for 18 years. They were companions. When SuSu died in 1998, Carl, someone who never seemed to get sick, almost immediately fell ill with a bad cold.

Is there a connection, then, between pets and feeling good? We think so.

Animal Attraction

Our primitive ancestors began to domesticate animals some 10,000 years B.C. Nowadays, according to a survey published by the National Institutes of Health in the late 1980s, more than half of all U.S. households serve as home for at least one animal. Americans have more pets than children. Across the country, we have some 51 million dogs, 56 million cats, 45 million birds, 75 million other small mammals and reptiles (everything from hamsters, guinea pigs, and mice to geckos, lizards, and snakes), and millions of fish.

Why? What is the mutual attraction between beast and human? Part of it must be the desire of a higher life form to tame the wild kingdom and conquer the beast; another part, perhaps, is the interest in communicating and interacting with other, almost alien, otherworldly living beings. Closer to our immunological hearts, though, the attraction also stems from the need for companionship and the need to give and receive affection. Pets are our friends. We talk to them, touch them, play with them. They make us laugh. They make us feel wanted. And they love us without condition. Such factors have a tremendous impact on our psyches and perhaps our immune systems. We don't consciously know it, but pets, in short, may help keep us healthy. That BEWARE OF DOG sign in the yard scares away far more than would-be intruders. Your pet's mere presence may also ward off disease.

Pets and Health: Dr. Feelgood Meets Dr. Doolittle

Florence Nightingale, whose love, care and concern for the sick in the late 1800s served as the foundation for our modern-day nursing profession, recommended that bedridden invalids keep a caged bird nearby to help preserve health and speed recovery. She understood intuitively what medicine now understands physiologically and psychologically: People who interact with animals are healthier than those who do not. From high blood pressure, postsurgical recovery, blindness, physical rehabilitation, inactivity, and fatigue, to loneliness, stress, depression, and general emotional difficulties, a whole new field of pet-assisted therapy has emerged to help people with numerous physical, psychological, and social problems.

Introducing pets in in-patient and long-term care settings elevates disposition and sense of humor, facilitates communication, and considerably improves psychiatric symptoms of all kinds, according to a 1987 study dubbed Project Pup that was conducted in several Florida nursing homes (see "The Ark Drops Anchor in 'Eden'" on

The Ark Drops Anchor in "Eden"

Despite great strides of late, nursing homes and assisted-living hospices still can be relatively antiseptic, unhappy places. For their elderly residents, they are more like hospitals, not homes. A refreshing concept, though, has been sweeping the field. Residents do not consist entirely of sick, aging people. They also include dogs, cats, and birds. They're not just occasional visitors; they're full-time, round-the-clock residents.

The Eden Alternative is a fascinating approach to standard nursing home practices, designed to help nursing-home residents cope a little better with their situations. Designed by William H. Thomas, M.D., a physician in upstate New York and author of *Life Worth Living*, the concept includes not only pets but also plants and visits from children. This approach and others like it are cropping up in nursing homes across the country.

Ferns and fun-loving kids are fine, but the pet component of the Eden Alternative is both innovative and influential. A sheepdog wagging its tail as you get off an elevator and a couple of cats sauntering along the hallways are two comforting ways to be greeted as you are whisked about via wheelchair in a nursing home. The bright chirping of birds brings the briskness of daybreak into the afternoon.

The effect, though, is more than atmospheric. Preliminary research shows strikingly that the presence of pets benefits health. According to Dr. Thomas, nursing homes with pets in their environs have residents who rely less on medications, fall sick less frequently, have fewer infections, and generally are happier than their counterparts in facilities that lack animal friendships.

This is natural immunity in action. Dogs, cats, and birds do not cure old age or Alzheimer's disease. They do, however, improve the environment and keep people feeling and thinking healthier.

page 124). Another investigation found that the presence of birds at group-therapy sessions encouraged better attendance and participation, diminished hostility, and hastened discharge from the forum. And older people who own pets spend less money on health care as compared with nonowners; they spend less time in the hospital, too, according to another study. Dog owners of all ages get more exercise, socialize in public more frequently, and even smile more often.

Petting Your Psyche

As goes the physiological, so goes the psychological. Another whole host of studies revealed the psychological and overall health benefits of having a pet. A 1991 British study at the University of Cambridge, for instance, followed 71 people who recently purchased a cat or dog and compared their psychological and physical health with that of a similar group of people who did not have animals. Pet owners displayed a general improvement in their overall psychological profiles and, within a month of adopting Rover or Tabby, fewer minor health nuisances. This remained so for the first 6 months of the study. For some reason, only dog owners showed a consistent, persistent improvement in health over the entire 10-month study period. Dog owners, compared with those who had cats, also displayed an increase in self-esteem and a reduction in anxiety over becoming a crime victim. They got more exercise, too.

The next time you're sweating over Form 1040 and Schedule C, you better have the dog at your feet or the cat in your lap. As a 1999 study at the State University of New York School of Medicine in Buffalo demonstrated, pet owners add, subtract, multiply, and divide better when the animals are present in the room. The study's scientists, according to a 1999 paper delivered in Prague at the Eighth Annual International Conference on Human-Animal Interaction, subjected a group to some mental arithmetic, a known stress inducer. When their pets were with them, the people performed better and reacted more calmly, as evidenced by blood pressure readings and heart rate.

In case we (or the medical literature) seem biased in favor of

Feline and Canine Cardiologists

A solid body of scientific research, along with more anecdotal studies, supports the contention that the presence of pets helps your heart. One of the very first systematic attempts to assess the influence of pets on health was a U.S. federal government Public Health Report published in 1980 that examined year-later survival rates of 82 people who were admitted to a hospital coronary care unit in the 1970s for either coronary-related chest pains (angina pectoris) or a heart attack. Among heart patients who did not own pets, 28 percent died in the following year, while only 6 percent of pet-owning patients passed away. The survival difference among those who did or did not own pets persisted independent of the severity of the heart condition.

The conclusion remains striking even today. Upon publication, questions emerged immediately, including, among other things, whether study participants might have benefited indirectly from the exercise gained by walking a dog. As it turned out, however, the speculation proved to be unfounded. Even those who owned pets other than pooches enjoyed the 1-year survival advantage. So strong was the association, that this study led in following years to numerous other investigations emphasizing animal companionship and contact comfort on cardiovascular risk factors. Petting a dog, these research ef-

dogs and, to a lesser extent, cats, note that a plethora of other studies demonstrates physical and psychological benefits no matter what pet you prefer. Riding a horse, for example, improves socialization and the effectiveness of psychotherapy (as well as, among people with movement disorders, posture, balance, mobility, and function), according to a trio of separate German studies conducted in 1976, 1981, and 1991. And a small 1988 study of eight males between the ages of 12 and 25 illustrated that some people with autism behaved better socially and had longer attention spans if they spent time with dolphins. (This is interesting but has not been scientifically replicated.)

forts demonstrated, reduces blood pressure, pulse, and respiratory rate in both children and adults. Equally important, mere tactile stimulation is not solely responsible. If you own or know the animal, a 1983 investigation of coronary and long-term care patients showed that the improvement in cardiac vital signs is even more dramatic.

Other research found that sometimes simply petting the dog is more beneficial than petting it and talking to it simultaneously. Why might this be so? While "getting it off your chest" generally is helpful, research does show that at certain times the simple act of talking actually elevates blood pressure. If, for instance, you visit your Uncle Ralph, chances are you're not going to just sit there in silence. At some point, you'll feel like you must say something. With Rover, you need not say a word if you don't feel like it. Silence is golden with a retriever, not a relative.

The research continues to this day. For example, a 1991 study of 6,000 men and women older than 40 conducted at the Baker Medical Institute in Melbourne, Australia, concluded that owning a pet lowers not only blood pressure but also triglycerides and cholesterol. The scientists could not attribute the better cardiovascular profiles to other lifestyle factors. The only clearly responsible difference was whether or not a person owned a pet.

Our Research: Petting and Other Plush Pleasures

The psychological and physiological variables in the body of research we encountered intrigued us. A mind-body, neurological-immunological interaction theoretically could exist between health and pet ownership. Jasmine, a cute little sheltie, soon became a frequent visitor and distinguished research colleague as we began to test the effect of her presence on study participants' immunoglobulin A (IgA) levels.

Two saliva tests, one taken immediately before each of 10 participants interacted with Jasmine and another immediately after an 18-minute petting session, should provide a good indication. In case personal preference came into play, we ruled out any participant who disliked dogs. To make sure that nothing else might account for any IgA change, we added a control group of 6 participants who sat in a room for the same period of time without any contact. Finally, to test the possibility that any tactile stimulation (scientific language for "touch") might influence IgA, we commissioned the creation of a stuffed replica of Jasmine, which would be petted and stroked for 18 minutes by each of the 9 individuals in yet another group. We now had all the bases covered. The only thing we would not learn is how all the affection and attention would influence Jasmine's immune system. (We assume it exerted an enormously positive influence.)

So what happened? The students who sat on the sofa in our test room without any contact with the sheepdog showed no increase in IgA. Students who spent time with Jasmine displayed an IgA elevation of about 12 percent. Those who petted Jasmine's stuffed replica also enjoyed an IgA boost, although to a lesser extent (about 7 percent). Obviously, touching anything soft and cuddly, whether alive or inanimate, positively sways immune strength. The greater IgA increase among those who interacted with the real Jasmine suggests something, but the results don't fully indicate what it all means. We never formally published the results of this pilot study, but its lingering questions, along with media interest in our findings (including a visit to our lab by noted British TV personality Angela Lamont and a producer from the British Broadcasting Corporation) prompted us to pursue further the pet connection to immune health.

More Research, Better Results

For our next experiment, begun in 1999, we followed the same general procedure as in the initial Jasmine study, albeit with a few important differences. For one, we almost doubled the number of participants, up to 55—an adequate number to assess the statistical reliability of the eventual findings. For another, we did not immediately exclude anyone with an aversion to pets. Instead, we administered, just before the 18-minute petting session, something called the Pet Attitude Scale, a survey that assesses how much a person likes or dislikes animals.

This time out, the results were more intriguing.

◆ The people who sat alone quietly showed no change in IgA. We suspected as much, because they sunk themselves into a comfortable, cushy couch that likely promoted relaxation.

◆ Those who squeezed and stroked the impostor Jasmine also showed an IgA increase, but again, one not statistically significant.

◆ Students who petted the authentic Jasmine, no matter what their professed attitude toward animals, did enjoy a substantial, statistically significant IgA elevation, one that validates our earlier study's findings.

Analyzing results of the Pet Attitude Scale enabled us to put the IgA results into better context.

Was the IgA increase in any way related to an individual's general disposition toward pets? No—at least not for people who sat alone on the sofa or for those who petted the real Jasmine. Among students who petted the stuffed replica, however, a quite high, statistically significant correlation did exist between their affinity for animals and their increases in IgA. Stated another way, people who generally like dogs, cats, birds, and other pets might improve their immune health simply by hugging an inanimate representation of the animal. Those who are less predisposed to animals will not benefit immunologically.

Allow us to explain in more detail: For 4 out of the 19 participants in the no-contact group, and for 3 out of 19 people in the Jasmine group, IgA actually declined—attributable to any of myriad external, extraneous variables. In other words, these people could have had something else weighing on their minds: a spat with a lover, a flunked philosophy exam, or an overdue credit card bill.

(continued on page 132)

Your Animal Instincts

This Pet Attitude Scale, developed by Dr. Donald I. Templer, a psychologist at the Psychological Services Center in Fresno, California, and his colleagues, is the one we used in our studies of the immune benefits on people who petted and stroked a plush stuffed dog. To find out what your likelihood of immune system benefit is based on our data, take the test yourself.

Answer each of the following questions as honestly as you can in terms of how you feel right now. Don't worry about how you think others might answer these questions—there aren't any right or wrong answers. All that matters is that you express your true feelings on the subject.

Circle one of the seven numbers for each question. When doing this, you'll notice that the points for questions 4, 6, 9, 12, 13, 15, and 17 are reversed; this is intentional. (For example, a rating of "strongly disagree" on question number 4 receives a "7" rather than a "1," while "moderately disagree" is "6" rather than "2.")

1. I really like seeing pets enjoy their food.

1	2	3	4	5	6	7
strongly disagree	moderately disagree	slightly disagree	unsure	slightly agree	moderately agree	strongly agree

2. My pet means more to me than any of my friends.

1	2	3	4	5	6	7
strongly disagree	moderately disagree	slightly disagree	unsure	slightly agree	moderately agree	strongly agree

3. I would like a pet in my own home.

1	2	3	4	5	6	7
strongly disagree	moderately disagree	slightly disagree	unsure	slightly agree	moderately agree	strongly agree

4. Having pets is a waste of money.

7	6	5	4	3	2	1
strongly disagree	moderately disagree	slightly disagree	unsure	slightly agree	moderately agree	strongly agree

5. House pets add happiness to my life (or would if I had one).

1	2	3	4	5	6	7
strongly disagree	moderately disagree	slightly disagree	unsure	slightly agree	moderately agree	strongly agree

6. I feel that pets should always be kept outside.

7	6	5	4	3	2	1
strongly disagree	moderately disagree	slightly disagree	unsure	slightly agree	moderately agree	strongly agree

7. I spend time every day playing with my pet (or would if I had one).

1	2	3	4	5	6	7
strongly disagree	moderately disagree	slightly disagree	unsure	slightly agree	moderately agree	strongly agree

8. I have occasionally communicated with my pet and understood what it was trying to express.

1	2	3	4	5	6	7
strongly disagree	moderately disagree	slightly disagree	unsure	slightly agree	moderately agree	strongly agree

9. The world would be a better place if people would stop spending so much time caring for their pets and started caring more for other human beings instead.

7	6	5	4	3	2	1
strongly disagree	moderately disagree	slightly disagree	unsure	slightly agree	moderately agree	strongly agree

10. I like to feed animals out of my hand.

1	2	3	4	5	6	7
strongly disagree	moderately disagree	slightly disagree	unsure	slightly agree	moderately agree	strongly agree

11. I love pets.

1	2	3	4	5	6	7
strongly disagree	moderately disagree	slightly disagree	unsure	slightly agree	moderately agree	strongly agree

12. Animals belong in the wild or in zoos, but not in the home.

7	6	5	4	3	2	1
strongly disagree	moderately disagree	slightly disagree	unsure	slightly agree	moderately agree	strongly agree

(continued)

Your Animal Instincts (cont.)

13. If you keep pets in the house, you can expect a lot of damage to furniture.

7	6	5	4	3	2	1
strongly disagree	moderately disagree	slightly disagree	unsure	slightly agree	moderately agree	strongly agree

14. I like house pets.

1	2	3	4	5	6	7
strongly disagree	moderately disagree	slightly disagree	unsure	slightly agree	moderately agree	strongly agree

15. Pets are fun, but it's not worth the trouble of owning one.

7	6	5	4	3	2	1
strongly disagree	moderately disagree	slightly disagree	unsure	slightly agree	moderately agree	strongly agree

16. I frequently talk to my pet.

1	2	3	4	5	6	7
strongly disagree	moderately disagree	slightly disagree	unsure	slightly agree	moderately agree	strongly agree

17. I hate animals.

7	6	5	4	3	2	1
strongly disagree	moderately disagree	slightly disagree	unsure	slightly agree	moderately agree	strongly agree

18. You should treat your house pets with as much respect as you would a human member of your family.

1	2	3	4	5	6	7
strongly disagree	moderately disagree	slightly disagree	unsure	slightly agree	moderately agree	strongly agree

Among the stuffed-dog participants who liked pets less than others, 7 out of 17 (about 41 percent) showed an IgA decline, a ratio too high to attribute to chance or statistical accident.

Statistically, what this means is that a significant relationship exists between one's attitude toward pets and IgA changes measured while interacting with a stuffed animal. The less you like our four-

Interpreting Your Score

Add the total number of points that you received for the 18 questions. Your total will range somewhere between 18 and 126 and will fall into one of our defined categories. While these categories certainly can't be carved in stone, we made some estimates of immune system benefit based solely on our sample. The category delineations were created using the mean, median, standard deviation, and estimate of standard error for the group who petted the stuffed dog, because this was the group that showed differences in benefit based on scores on the Pet Attitude Scale. (Our research suggests that when a live animal is involved, you're likely to benefit regardless of your score on this scale.)

If your score was . . .	Your likelihood of benefit is . . .
in the 120s	You're about certain to benefit from stuffed animals. In fact, if the effects are conditioned responses, a picture of your favorite pet might do it.
115–120	You're likely to benefit from stroking a stuffed animal. Make it a replica of your favorite pet, if possible.
90–115	Benefits here are a coin flip. Odds increase greatly above a score of 108.
80–90	You need the real thing.
in the 70s or below	Have sex, eat chocolate, or listen to your favorite CD instead of stroking a stuffed animal.

footed friends, the more likely your immune defenses will either drop or remain unchanged when stroking a stuffed dog doll; the more you like animals, the more likely your IgA will jump up while cuddling a stuffed dog.

To recap, statistical analyses demonstrated two things: First, you do not have to be favorably disposed to animals to benefit from their

When a Pet Dies

Have you ever visited a pet cemetery? They often are awe-inspiring places, dotted with expensive marble headstones and elaborate, personalized shrines that feature photographs, favored toys, and chewed-up slippers.

If you've ever had a dog, cat, bird, or other pet, loss of the animal, no matter how long you shared your life with it, can strike you as hard as the loss of a spouse or a child. Should you get another pet? If so, how soon? Well, that depends. Generally, though, we recommend getting a new animal companion as soon as possible, with one caveat: Understand that a new pet is not a replacement companion; rather, it's a different companion. Preserve the memory of your lost loved one, but enjoy the pleasure of your new pet.

Do not act too hastily, though. Think about the implications. Sometimes, people cannot overcome the guilt. If you cannot move beyond this point, consider a different type of pet that will not be a direct reminder of the faithful companion you lost. If it still feels too uncomfortable, wait, but keep the door open. Let a little more time pass and assess your feelings again. Given the state of our current lifestyles, you might decide that you just cannot accept the responsibility. When Carl's SuSu died, for example, he and his wife decided that getting another dog was too much like having a baby at that point in their lives.

If you ultimately choose to not get another pet, please go out of your way to insert other pleasures into your life. Laugh a little more. Listen to music a little more. Cuddle a little more.

---

presence. Among the students who petted the real Jasmine, most benefited immunologically no matter what their attitude toward pets. Second, if you like animals, you're going to enjoy an immune system boost simply by stroking a plush facsimile. Is this attributable to the tactile stimulation or to the positive feelings associated with the resemblance to a beloved critter? We suggest a combination of both—another instance in which personal preference enters into the formula.

This is Pavlovian conditioning in action: A neutral object takes on a positive or negative charge simply by its association in your mind with something that automatically elicits positive or negative emotions.

Getting Connected . . .
with Animal Instincts

Dog, cat, canary, cockatoo, horse, hamster, fish, ferret, rabbit, mouse, lizard, iguana, chameleon, snake, pig, chicken, goat—it doesn't matter. The bottom line is simple and direct: If you like pets, get one and interact with it. The interaction is what is most important. The more you connect with the animal world, the more your immune system benefits. Part of the advantage is a direct connection between you and your favorite animal. Another part is the Pavlovian conditioning that you've come to expect by seeing a particular animal and the general conditioning that your mind has come to know just by interacting with and experiencing animals.

How might you benefit immunologically from the animal world? We have several additional suggestions that might not be immediately apparent.

Strike a consensus. Get a pet that the whole family enjoys. If Mom hates dogs and Dad hates cats, a cat or a dog probably is not the best pet to get. From person to person, animals generate widely divergent emotional reactions. Sit down, talk about what pet best suits the household. Come to a calm, mutually acceptable agreement. If this little friend is not welcomed wholeheartedly by the entire family, the immune enhancement won't fully work.

Love the one you're with. Acquiring a pet is similiar to having a baby. If you cannot attend to the responsibilities, if you are not up to the task, then don't do it. It's not fair to the animal. We've all heard stories about neglected pets that fall ill, either physically or psychologically or both. You may have seen video footage on TV of unresponsive dogs that sit trembling in warm cages as if shivering, or know of birds that self-destructively pluck out their own feathers. These animals have suffered major emotional damage because they have not been properly cared for and loved.

It goes both ways. Animals also may be sensitive to the presence or absence of pleasure, attention, and affection. Ever wonder why the pet you loved the most seemed to live the longest? Perhaps it's because you stoked the little thing's immunological fires.

Enjoy the demands. The more a pet relies on you for its existence and good health, the more you feel needed. The more you feel needed, the more you'll feel that you have a purpose in life, and that's a big benefit for you.

Get Pavlov on your side. We are not suggesting that you buy a dog that salivates whenever the doorbell rings. What we mean is that Pavlov's conditioning principle can work to your immunological advantage (or disadvantage) when selecting a pet. In other words, you probably are predisposed, either positively or negatively, to certain animals. If, when you were a child, the neighbor's Doberman scared you half to death each time you walked by it, don't get a Doberman. (In fact, you may have cultivated a fear and aversion to dogs in general.) If, however, you recall fond memories of your favorite aunt every time you see a poodle, you certainly should consider getting a poodle. If a classic orange tabby was your constant companion when you were young, a similar-looking cat is a good pet to get now.

Pick your pleasure. Which are better, cats or dogs? Ah, a perennial battle. We may risk some wrath here, but if in doubt about what pet to get—if you do not care one way or the other—get a dog. A dog is very faithful. It is more likely to attend to your needs, inadvertently supporting your immune health. (Most research on the health benefits of having a pet has focused on our canine friends. Most self-esteem studies with animals, too, have concentrated on dog ownership.)

If you simply do not like dogs or can't see yourself walking and cleaning up after one, get a cat. The cat will take to you, but on its own terms. Remember, although she may act more self-reliant, Tabby needs you just as much as a dog would.

The word about birds (or lizards or guinea pigs or any other caged pets). Birds, you might be surprised to know, like to be scratched just like dogs and petted just like cats. So do ferrets, chameleons, turtles, and frogs. Science has determined that birds can not only mimic human speech, but they can also remember faces from the past. Toads do amazing things too. Do not rule out any animal friend, but rather assess your predilections honestly.

Share in the care. Once the whole household agrees on a pet, the whole household should share in the care and enjoyment of this little wonder. Everyone should feed it. Everyone should fondle it. The interaction will increase communication among family members, and that can only serve to boost immunity.

Don't get into rivalries. You'll no doubt eventually see that your pet likes everyone in your family in somewhat different ways. Sometimes the pet will aim right for you. At other times it will ignore you and head straight toward your spouse, your son, or your daughter. It may even sulk off and ignore the whole lot of you. Do not feel slighted. Revel in these interactive differences and curiosities. They are signs that you and your family are interacting with another intelligent, sensitive being that has his own emotional preferences, and different moods and wants, at different times of the day and night.

Talk to the animals. Look in your pet's eyes and talk to it. You will see a reaction. You will see a direct connection and a hint of understanding. Bare your craziest secrets, your most embarrassing moments, your doubts and most horrible shortcomings. Say whatever you want to say. Get it all off your chest and you will end up much better, psychologically and immunologically. Your pet will not care about what you divulge. Your pet will still love you. And it won't tell another living soul.

Let them entertain you. From the dog that catches Frisbees and the cat that goes to the bathroom in the toilet to the bird that whistles "The Star-Spangled Banner," we know that pets are capable of all sorts of wacky antics. We know, too, how immunologically important it is to smile and laugh. It's another synergy of pleasures for better immune protection.

Go for a stroll. Dogs are the best pets to help you get some immune-boosting exercise. Many people, however, also put leashes on their cats and take them for walks. Some pet stores that specialize in our avian friends even sell leashes for such bigger birds as cockatoos and macaws.

Give your parents a pet. You likely would not have known the joy of living with a pet had it not been for your mom and dad. Presumably, they too appreciate the life and love that animals offer. If you are ever faced with the difficult choice of entering a parent into a nursing home or assisted-living center, consider a facility whose residents include dogs, cats, and birds.

Cuddle up with a counterfeit. If you cannot, for whatever reason, snuggle with a real Rover or Fluffy, swallow your pride, ignore the embarrassment, and get a stuffed animal or two. The plush counterparts are more than children's toys and shooting-gallery prizes at carnivals. They serve as pillows and decorative home accents with a positive immunity impact. Its effects are less pronounced than when you're hugging the real thing, but nonetheless you'll benefit big-time if you like animals.

Go to the zoo. The immune system may benefit from the mere presence of animals, even if they are behind bars and unreachable. Plan a morning or afternoon outing with family or a friend at the zoo. Alternatively, find a local bird-watching group and become a member to better appreciate their dawn-breaking sights and sounds.

Aim an eye on the kingdom. Knowing what we know from the previous chapter about the significant immunity impact of just viewing an enjoyable movie or TV show, spend some of your channel-hopping time on the Animal Planet cable station. It regularly features heartwarming programs about our fuzzy, furry, and feathered friends, along with funny, inspiring, in-depth profiles of exotic creatures from around the world. The shows demonstrate that animals really are not all that different from us, and that knowledge can really help nurture us as we identify with their behaviors and struggles.

Similarly, rent one of the many movies in which the star walks on four legs. For starters, try *Bambi* and *Old Yeller*, both definite tear-jerkers. For laughs, try *That Darn Cat*. For love, rent *Lady and the Tramp*. For inspiration, go back to *Born Free*. And for pure sentimental sweetness, humor, and Oscar-winning special effects, watch *Babe*, the 1996 Golden Globe winner for best comedy or musical, about a sheepherding pig and his barnyard friends.

Get along, little digitized doggie. Everyone needs a screensaver for his computer. Why not put your favorite animal on your monitor? After returning to your desk from a long meeting, a testy one-on-one with your boss, or even a pleasant coffee break, wouldn't it be nice (and immunologically inspiring) to be greeted by the happy face of a favorite animal?

Go to the wall. Similarly, decorate the walls of your home with pictures of your favorite animals. No, we do not recommend one of those velvet paintings of dogs playing poker. We do, though, suggest that you obtain a few photographs or paintings of animals to hang on the wall in various rooms of your home.

Chapter 7

Humor

It Really Is the Best Medicine

A merry heart doeth good like a medicine;
but a broken spirit drieth the bones.
—Proverbs 17:22

Doctors finally diagnosed why Norman was in so much agony—agony that rendered him virtually incapable of lying down, resting, and turning over without resorting to painkillers, let alone standing up and moving about. He had ankylosing spondylitis, an incurable degenerative rheumatic disease that inflames and stiffens joints in the spinal cord and thorax.

Norman had, according to the best medical estimates, about 3 months left to live. Get your affairs in order, his physicians advised.

Chemotherapy and radiation treatments were doctors' orders, but Norman rejected that advice. He had several other obvious options, but he chose none of them. He did not turn to religion in his waning days in search of a miraculous cure or to atone for his evil ways. He did not become a drinking, partying, carousing hedonist in a last-ditch effort to live life to the fullest. Nor did he lapse into a deep depression and resign himself to his diagnosed fate. We are talking about Norman Cousins, the esteemed, long-time editor of the prestigious *Saturday Review* and author of *Anatomy of an Illness*, who beat the odds and overcame an incurable illness with, apparently, not much more than a bunch of belly laughs.

Die Laughing? Hah!

Cousins was diagnosed and handed his 3-month death sentence in 1964, at the age of 39. After reading Hans Selye's groundbreaking research linking stress to health, he decided to go for broke and test the long-held *Reader's Digest* proposition that laughter really is the best medicine. He began a daily diet of Marx Brothers movies, Three Stooges shorts, and episodes of *Candid Camera*. (He also took a lot of vitamin C.) After just 10 minutes of laughing himself silly, Cousins soon noticed that he could sleep without pain and without need for medication for up to 2 hours. Even the doctors noted that after a hearty laugh, inflammation in Cousins's body, for reasons they could not explain, lessened.

The 3-month deadline came . . . and went. Cousins did not die. As the daily chucklefests continued for the next 3 months, the *Saturday Review* editor was still both alive and well! Ankylosing spondylitis was no longer ravaging his body. The disease had remitted entirely.

More than a decade later, in 1979, a still-healthy Cousins recounted his ordeal and his recovery in the book *Anatomy of an Illness*. He also became an adjunct professor in the department of behavioral medicine at the University of California, Los Angeles, School of Medicine, where he established a humor task force to promote and coordinate research into laughter's impact on health. Later, UCLA's AIDS Institute created the Norman Cousins Program in Psychoneuroimmunology to fund both PNI research and doctoral training. Cousins remained an advocate of mind-body medicine for the rest of his life. He had his last laugh in 1990, when he died at the ripe age of 75.

Funny Pharmacy and Madcap Medicine?

Could Cousins's remission have been completely unrelated to his humor therapy? Absolutely. Diseases remit spontaneously all the time for reasons unknown. Cousins was one man, and his chronicles in no way, shape, or form represent a scientifically conducted experiment. Could his remarkable, inexplicable recovery be attributable, even in part, to laughter and positive emotions? Again, absolutely. He believed it could. So do we.

In the 1960s and 1970s, Cousins's groundbreaking notion went unsupported by even a shred of medical evidence. Today, though, a body of scientific research sustains the proposition that the funny bone is connected to the immune bone.

Let a Smile Be Your (Immunological) Umbrella

In the aftermath of publicity generated by Cousins's remission and recovery, researchers began to subject his claims to scientific scrutiny. In one early investigation, a small 1985 study headed by Kathleen Dillon, Ph.D., a psychologist at Western New England College in Springfield, Massachusetts, 4 men and 6 women first watched a half-hour of video showing Richard Pryor performing live, then another 30 minutes of a neutral, humor-free video. By the time they had finished laughing along with Pryor, the study participants' immunoglobulin A (IgA) measurements had risen 20 percent. After viewing the neutral tape, their IgA levels had not budged. Dr. Dillon and her colleagues did not stop there, though. They administered to the 10 study participants a questionnaire designed to elicit whether or not they used humor to deal with problems in their lives. Those who tended to employ humor as a coping mechanism had higher initial IgA readings.

(continued on page 146)

Two Thumbs Up: Movies and TV Shows That Will Tickle Your Funny Bone

In the spring of 2000, the venerable American Film Institute issued its list of the top 100 funniest movies of all time. *Some Like It Hot*, featuring the cross-dressing team of Jack Lemmon and Tony Curtis, topped the roster, followed by such notables as *Tootsie, Dr. Strangelove, Annie Hall, Duck Soup, Blazing Saddles, M*A*S*H, It Happened One Night, The Graduate*, and *Airplane!* The list can be found at www.afionline.org.

For weeks and weeks, the list was a wonderful conversation starter and argument instigator at home and at work. We, as observers of both the psyche and the silly, don't agree with all of the selections. While all of the movies at the top of the list certainly are amusing, except for two of them we think we've seen far funnier flicks. As a public health service, both mentally and immunologically, we offer our own highly subjective picks for not only the funniest movies ever made but also the funniest TV shows ever broadcast. Here they are, in no particular preferential order.

Film Funnies

Airplane! One of the dumbest and funniest movies of all time, it spoofs the disaster movies of the 1970s. Leslie Nielsen steals the show as a doctor on board the ill-fated flight. "You'd better tell the captain we've got to land as soon as we can. This woman has to be gotten to a hospital!" he orders stewardess Julie Hagerty. "A hospital?! What is it?" she exclaims, wanting to know what is wrong with the ailing woman. "It's a big building with patients," Nielsen replies.

Austin Powers: The Spy Who Shagged Me. As he readily acknowledges, Powers put the *grrrr* in "swinger." Mike Myers, another *Saturday Night Live* alumnus, spoofs 1960s spy movies and the whole psychedelic era, from clothing to music to attitude. "How do you get into those pants?" Powers quizzes the alluring Felicity Shagwell about her skintight, seemingly painted-on clothing. "Well," she replies, "you can start by buying me a drink."

Caddyshack. A movie ostensibly about golf, but the links serve only as a backdrop for all other matters of hilarity. "I'm no slouch, you know," Ted Knight's character asserts to Chevy Chase. "Don't be so hard on yourself,

Judge," Chase responds with sympathy and reassurance. "You're a tremendous slouch."

Duck Soup. A classic Marx Brothers romp from 1933 that stands the test of time with a riotous, nonstop succession of unforgettable sight gags and pun-filled dialogue. At one point, Chico is promised "seven years in Leavenworth—or eleven years in Sevenworth," to which he replies, "I'll take five and ten at Woolworth's."

Ghostbusters. Who else are you gonna call other than Bill Murray and company when a gigantic otherworldly Pillsbury Doughboy look-alike wreaks havoc in a major metropolis? It's a funny movie with classic dialogue, good special effects, and a snappy title tune.

History of the World, Part I. The comic genius who helped give us the 2,000-Year-Old Man returns with a bawdy, racy review of life on Earth since the beginning of time. As emperor Comicus, Brooks notes that, "The only thing we Romans don't have a god for is premature ejaculation. But I hear that's coming quickly."

The Naked Gun. Leslie Nielsen graduated from physician in *Airplane!* to police detective Lieutenant Frank Drebin in this equally wacky series of cop-movie spoofs.

National Lampoon's *Vacation*. Chevy Chase takes his dysfunctionally normal family on a do-or-die trek to Wally World, a theme park. The family eventually does succeed, but not without a hilarious mishap every minute of the way. Why did they drive instead of fly? As Chevy explains in the movie, "Because getting there is half the fun."

The Pink Panther. The first of a fine series of madcap movies starring the irrepressible Peter Sellers as Inspector Jacques Clouseau. "What kind of bomb was planted?" someone asks the canny French detective. "The exploding kind," Sellers deadpans.

Tommy Boy. The late Chris Farley portrays a lovable imbecile trying to save his family's business with the help of pal David Spade, fellow *Saturday Night Live* alumnus. It's a good farce.

(continued)

Two Thumbs Up: Movies and TV Shows That Will Tickle Your Funny Bone (cont.)

Televised Tickles

The Bob Newhart Show. Dr. Bob Hartley, a Chicago psychologist, was a perfect vehicle for the straight-faced, deadpan humor of the legendary Bob Newhart. We're favorably disposed just because he was a psychologist. You should be favorably disposed because he, his wife, his friends, and his patients were just plain funny.

Cheers. Should everybody know your name? Why not? We all know the names of Sam, Diane, Frasier, Norm, Cliffy, and Carla. And we're glad they came onto the TV screen.

M*A*S*H. War might be hell, but don't you wish you had the chance to hang out at the 4077th Mobile Army Surgical Hospital? Fans may debate whether the earlier, loonier episodes were funnier than the later shows filled with more righteous indignation; but Hawkeye, Trapper, B. J., Henry, Colonel Potter, Margaret, Frank, Charles, Radar, Klinger, and Father Mulcahy consistently used humor, irony, and just plain insanity to drive home the horrible inhumanity of war—and the healing, coping force of laughing in the face of death. Other TV shows might be inherently funnier, but perhaps none other made a more poignant, better case for buffering stress and adversity with humor.

Seinfeld. Jerry, Elaine, George, and Kramer in 1990s New York City. Soup Nazi, a cigar-store Indian, a run-amok children's party, a dead bird, George's accidentally killed fiancée—yadda, yadda, yadda. It's funny. Watch it.

By the dawn of the following decade, the connection between humor and immunity had become more strongly documented, thanks in part to the work of Herbert Lefcourt, Ph.D., a psychologist at the University of Waterloo in Canada. In a 1990 paper, Lefcourt detailed results of three humor-related studies. In the first, 45 female college students laughed along to an audiotape of the classic 2,000-Year-Old Man sketch performed by Mel Brooks and Carl Reiner. At the end of the skit, the women's IgA levels had risen, al-

The Simpsons. Not many other shows are so consistently funny on so many levels. Unlike *The Flintstones*, which was remarkably similar to Jackie Gleason's *The Honeymooners*, the creators of *The Simpsons* broke ground, and their cartoon characters served as the basis for other, lesser sitcoms with real people.

The Beauty of the Belly Laugh

But what about *I Love Lucy*? What about *All in the Family, Frasier,* and *Everybody Loves Raymond*? What about *Hee Haw* and *Monty Python's Flying Circus*? What about *This Is Spinal Tap, Moonstruck, The Nutty Professor, Abbott and Costello Meet Frankenstein,* anything with Woody Allen, and so many other uproarious movies and TV shows?

Well, that's the best part: Humor is entirely subjective. You cannot be wrong. Whatever you find funny is going to elevate your IgA and improve your defense against disease. It doesn't matter if two psychologists like it. Who are we to judge? Our taste in movies obviously runs toward idiotic slapstick anyway. We merely offer our suggestions as a launching pad. What matters is if *you* like it. *De gustibus non disputandum est* is the Latin dictum, and it translates into, "In matters of taste, there is no argument." As long as you like it, and it makes you laugh, it can be a contributor to your immune health.

beit not to the extent recorded in the Western New England College experiment. Perhaps the aural-only influence on immunity is less powerful than the audiovisual influence, at least when it comes to laughing?

Dr. Lefcourt and colleagues conducted further research, this time treating the audience to 30 minutes of the video *Bill Cosby, Himself.* Maybe the Cos is just funnier than Brooks and Reiner, because the test participants' immune systems responded by displaying IgA elevations comparable to those in the Western New England study. For good measure, the University of Waterloo researchers also administered a questionnaire designed to measure their study participants' sense of humor. Those with a bigger, better sense of humor showed more dramatic improvements in IgA upon watching Cosby. This makes intuitive sense: The more you appreciate the funny side of life, the more you will benefit.

America's Funniest?

Of all the scientific evidence attesting to the immunological improvement of laughter, three studies in particular demonstrate different aspects of the proposition.

◆ In 1995 a research duo from Arkansas Tech University in Russellville, Roy Lambert, R.N., and Nancy Lambert, R.N., wondered whether kids also benefited immunologically from humor. They gathered 39 fifth-graders, turned on the TV and the VCR, and let them watch segments of *America's Funniest Home Videos*, mostly home movies of newlyweds falling into wedding cakes, dads taking unexpected dips in the backyard pool, and babies being tackled by the family pooch. The 39 kids liked what they saw: Their IgA levels rose significantly.

◆ If it's funny, you can't help but benefit. Ever try to suppress a laugh? Perhaps guffawing was inappropriate in the situation, such as when the boss said something ludicrously silly during a staff meeting. Perhaps you didn't want to contribute to the embarrassment of the object of your giggles, such as when your gravel-throated best friend thought he was the Caruso of karaoke with his rendition of "Feelings." Whether you laugh out loud or not doesn't matter, according to a study by Susan Labott, Ph.D., and colleagues at the University of Toledo in Ohio. The researchers sat down 39 female students and screened for them the video *Bill Cosby: 49*. The women were told either to be aware of and fully express their emotions, or to inhibit any desire to grin and chuckle. Whether they laughed openly or not, all of their IgA levels rose.

The immunological benefit, in other words, is beyond your control. If you wipe a smile off your face as you watch some hapless clod fall in a puddle of water—even if you're laughing on the inside but not outwardly—your immune system is laughing with you and benefiting you.

◆ In a study by Lesley Harrison, Ph.D., and colleagues at the University of Birmingham in England, 30 healthy undergraduate students, equally divided between males and females, watched three 10-minute movie clips designed to evoke different emotions. A stand-up comedy routine was designed to elicit laughter; a clip from the 1998 penalty shoot-out between England and Argentina in the World Cup was supposed to generate excitement; and a mathematics presentation was intended to serve as a neutral (if not boring) control. Interestingly, IgA rose after watching each of the tapes, regardless of content. Following a funny story, a bouncing ball, or a mathematical equation all seemed to carry the same immunological weight.

Well, not so fast. A few factors can account for the odd discrepancies with other research. First off, study participants viewed each film for only 10 minutes as opposed to a half-hour or more in the other experiments. Ten minutes may not be long enough for humor's immunological benefit to manifest itself fully. Moreover, the study participants watched the three clips within a relatively short 2-hour period. Even though an equal number of them saw the clips in each possible order, there still may have been some "contamination" from film to film that obscured any of humor's positive influence on IgA.

The most interesting aspect of the Birmingham study, though, is how watching the movies affected stress-related cardiovascular measurements. (This experiment foreshadows what you will learn in the ensuing section about why giggles make immune defenses grow.) The sporting event elevated viewers' blood pressure readings and heart rates, indicative of increased sympathetic (stress-provoked) nervous system activation. The comedy bit, in contrast, decreased blood pressure and cardiac output, which is associated with less stress and less sympathetic nervous system activity. Laughter, as should be no surprise, lessens stress and its potential for physiological damage.

The Merrier, The More

Science tends to focus on IgA as an immunity marker because it is, after all, the body's first line of defense against infection and illness, and because it is measured relatively easily. So don't think that humor does not tickle funny bones in other immunological parameters. In fact, there is other research, much of it conducted by Lee S. Berk, M.D., and his colleagues from the Loma Linda University School of Medicine in California. They have documented that chuckling, giggling, and guffawing also increase levels of IgM and IgG, two other immunoglobulins, as well as helper T cells, natural killer cells, and complement.

The Whys and Wherefores of Yuks

The simple fact is, laughter and a healthy sense of humor help you contend better with stress and its profound physiological effects.

We've all laughed ourselves to the point of almost total physical exhaustion. Perhaps it was over the flatulent bean-eating scene in *Blazing Saddles*. Maybe it was upon seeing a goofy grimace by Jim Carrey in *Ace Ventura: Pet Detective*. Or perhaps it was a recounting of an embarrassingly funny tale by a friend at a party. Whatever the impetus, your uncontrollable, unstoppable gigglefest accomplishes two things: It burns off calories, and it burns off stress chemicals.

You'll probably never lose a few waist sizes by laughing, but William Fry, M.D., professor emeritus at Stanford University School of Medicine, calculates that 100 consecutive laughs is aerobically equivalent to 15 minutes of peddling on a stationary bicycle. More important, however, is the exertion behind the laughter. It reduces muscle tension, he explains, and helps the body relax.

The resulting stress reduction is beneficial physiologically and emotionally no matter what the situation, according to Paul E. McGhee, Ph.D., a developmental psychologist who left years in academia to form the Laughter Remedy, a New Jersey firm that espouses the use of humor in any setting, from the corporate boardroom to the cancer ward.

Grin and Bear It (Better)

The better you roll with the punches and laugh off tension-generating problems, the less likely you will be negatively affected by adversity, according to the University of Waterloo's Dr. Lefcourt and colleague and fellow psychologist Rod Martin, Ph.D. The team has been responsible for much of the modern research into the relationship between humor and stress. In 1983 the two published a paper detailing the results of their Situational Humor Response Questionnaire, an 18-point survey of whether people would be amused in various scenarios, such as if you went to a party and saw someone wearing clothes identical to yours.

For people with a good sense of humor, negative events in their lives are not major disturbances. In contrast, people with a less-cultivated sense of humor are far more likely to be upset by negative events. Does the connection translate into stronger immunity? It does indeed, according to a later study by the Waterloo psychologists. After recounting the overall association between jocularity and the number 1 immunoglobulin, the researchers demonstrated that people with low positions on the humor totem pole had more pronounced declines in IgA when they encountered life's daily hassles. Laugh leaders experienced less of an IgA decrease.

The Martin-Lefcourt research strikes a powerful blow in favor of the humor-stress connection, stronger than the wallop that Bugs

Bunny packed when he loaded his glove with a horseshoe and slugged that burly boxer. If you recognize the humor in dark situations, your mood won't dip, and your IgA won't fall.

The Sledgehammer Effect

Need we further emphasize the influence of humor on stress reduction and immune fortification? Must we hit you on the head with a sledgehammer, a la the Three Stooges? Well, Dr. Berk and colleagues at Loma Linda University School of Medicine did incorporate a sledgehammer in their documentation of a specific, concrete, comedic decrease in stress chemicals.

Back in 1989 they recruited volunteers and had them either sit in silence for 60 minutes or view an hour-long video of Gallagher, the beret-wearing stand-up comic known for smashing watermelons (and other messy, splatter-prone objects) with a sledgehammer. Cortisol, a classic stress hormone, dropped in both groups, but it dipped farther for the folks who watched Gallagher. Those exposed to the comic's physical humor also had lower measurements of epinephrine and growth hormone, two other chemicals that reflect the body's response to stress by suppressing the immune system.

Do you need a sledgehammer to jar your immune system into action? We hope not. We presume that the reduction in cortisol, epinephrine, and other measures of stress is effected regardless of provocation. Slipping on a banana peel should be just as immunity enhancing as a hammer hit on the noggin.

Tears of a Clown: Sad Is Not So Bad

Linda Richman, the Mike Myers character on *Saturday Night Live* who hosted the "Coffee Talk" segment, often became weepily emotional. During attempts to regain her composure, she would give her audience a topic to talk over ("Rhode Island is neither a road nor an island. Discuss."). After her near-tears episodes, she always seemed to feel better, as did her laughing viewers.

Many women, although not many men, do report feeling better after a good cry. Some research links sobbing to immune suppression, however. For instance, the same University of Toledo study participants who watched Bill Cosby also watched a sentimentally sad video documenting a visit to a nursing home. Some were told to give full vent to their emotions, while others were told to hold back the tears. Among those who wept openly during the screening, IgA dropped. Not so for those who kept a stiff upper lip. Crying, it would appear, is bad for immune strength.

Do not jump to such a hasty conclusion, however. Timing seems to be everything.

We ran a similar study in which groups of study participants viewed 30 minutes of a sad movie. All participants indicated that they felt sad by what they saw. Those who maintained poker faces, with no tears, showed decreases in IgA. Those who sobbed displayed no change in IgA. The immune marker by no means increased, but it did not drop, either.

How, then, does this pertain to the discrepancy in the medical literature? We believe that it relates to when researchers measured IgA. Take the immunoglobulin levels and stress, for example. Experiments show that right around the time you first perceive the stressor, your IgA briefly rises. Soon after the initial elevation, though, it very predictably and definitely decreases. Crying may produce a similar, albeit inverse, situation: When the tears first start to flow, IgA levels may drop transiently, only to rebound and increase.

Clinical data and common sense suggest that a good cry is just that—good for you. Expressing emotion, whatever the emotion, is good for you. Even the venting of negative emotions provides an immunological lift, according to a series of experiments conducted in the 1990s by a team of researchers headed by Roger Booth, Ph.D., of the University of Auckland in New Zealand, and James Pennebaker, Ph.D., of the University of Texas at Austin. This transcontinental collaboration examined the immune effects of either expressing or suppressing emotions.

In one of the experiments, the scientists asked 65 medical students from Auckland University to sit down for 15 minutes and write about something either very emotional to them or something entirely neutral. Afterward, half of each group was told to think about their topics in detail; the other half of each group was instructed to put the incidents out of their minds entirely. This exercise was repeated for 3 consecutive days. Before and after each writing assignment, the researchers drew blood samples.

Among those who suppressed their thoughts, circulating T lymphocytes declined significantly whether or not the thoughts were emotionally laden. Giving vent to the thoughts contained in the writing, though, increased levels of T cells. The total number of lymphocytes also increased.

In and of themselves, these results are rather illuminating. But the breakthrough is, again, in the timing. Study participants wrote for 15 minutes and were told to mull over or to suppress their thoughts for just 5 minutes. Do the math, add up the results, and you will realize that the immune system's strength can change significantly in a mere 20 minutes.

The moral of the study is that suppressing thoughts, despite their content, is immunologically detrimental. It causes definite physiological shifts that probably relate to stress. Expressing any kind of emotion, even by writing about it, accelerates immune activity, while trying to repress it causes an immune system decline.

If something negative or painful is on your mind, then, give it free rein. Don't try to ignore it. In the end, it really does not go away. You know that. At some point you will have to confront it. As we have previously noted, women tend to be better at this than men. We have also noted that men, on average, die 6 years earlier than do women. We are not suggesting that this emotional tendency is the only element responsible for the longevity difference. We suspect, however, that it may be a contributing factor.

Getting Connected . . .
with Humor

Psychologically healthy people do not laugh all the time, nor should they. Some things are unquestionably sad and serious and should, overall, be addressed as such. Denial is not healthy either, so do not use a great sense of humor to avoid confronting troublesome situations. That proviso aside, we can now dispense our humorous horse pills.

Go for the jocular. Lighten up. Life throws absurdities in your face every single day. Sure, many if not all of them are infuriating, but if you saw them on a TV sitcom or in a movie, you'd laugh out loud at how preposterous the situation was. You would laugh not only at the provocation but at the steam-out-of-the-ears reaction of the hapless victim. *Catch-22* may be about the insanity of war, but it's also a pretty funny book. Do not dismiss the seriousness of any event, but do step outside of yourself, if only momentarily, and laugh at how ludicrous it is.

Rent and vent. Go to the neighborhood video store and browse the comedy section. Use the American Film Institute's list of top 100 funniest films of all time, or, as we would prefer in a more psychologically professional fashion, follow our own picks (see "Two Thumbs Up: Movies and TV Shows That Will Tickle Your Funny Bone" on pages 144–147). Or close your eyes, point, and take a chance. One way or the other, you will have at least a laugh or two or three. You'll get to second-guess the experts, you will stimulate conversation, and you will be entertained.

Let TV tickle. Television remains a source of big-time laughs. From Milton Berle, Lucy Ricardo, and Ralph Kramden to Archie Bunker, Hawkeye Pierce, and Mary Richards, from Sam and Cliffy to Rachel and Ross, TV is a treasure trove of laughter. Thanks to cable, you can sample everything from the oldest shows ever committed to tape to first runs of the newest sitcoms. Sit down on the sofa, grab the remote, and flip around. Chances are you will land on something that makes you laugh.

Move over to the movie theater. Where else can you pay seven bucks for three jujubes? If TV is not your cup of tea, go to the local theater complex. You get out of the house, you'll be with friends or a loved one, and you'll be entertained. Even the worst alleged comedy has an immunity-stimulating redeeming scene or two.

Talk it up. If you saw a funny movie over the weekend or watched a hilarious rerun of *Friends* the other evening, bring it up at work or the next party you attend. Initiate a discussion about humor and you will likely find yourself in the middle of a humorous discussion. Swap favorite lines and favorite gags. Even if you or your friends vociferously disagree, the interaction still will do everyone's immune systems a lot of good.

Live it up live. Every city of any size has at least one comedy club these days. Get some friends together and catch a stand-up act in person. You'll relax, enjoy the company, have a few drinks, and laugh. Unless you live in New York City or Los Angeles, chances are you will have never heard of the comedians or comediennes on stage, but you might several years later. Jay Leno, Jerry Seinfeld, Tim Allen, and Robin Williams are among many other big-name stars who got their starts as anonymous stand-up comedians on the comedy-club circuit.

Cry yourself a river. Sometimes sad is as good as silly. If you feel sad, be sad. When provoked, do not hesitate to shed a tear. Despite the divergence in medical literature, we believe that crying benefits both your emotional disposition and your immune system. Denying dark emotions will not make them go away. Don't dwell on them for too long, though. For one, they could become self-perpetuating, especially if your down mood generates a little more interest from family and friends. For another, those same friends and family members could grow a little tired of your moping.

Chapter 8

Light, Sight, and Insight

SEE THE LIGHT AND KEEP THE FAITH

Space and light and order. Those are the things that men need just as much as they need bread or a place to sleep.
—Le Corbusier, Swiss architect

Let there be light," it says in the book of Genesis. What a wonderful phrase, but what does the research say about light and the immune system? Light, or more technically, phototherapy, has been used for years to treat seasonal affective disorder, or SAD, a kind of depression common in the wintertime. Light has also been used as an adjunct therapy to improve the healing of wounds. (Light appears to help remove moisture from the wound and thus make the region less hospitable to microbes.)

Light is immunosuppressive, and thus seems to slow down the autoimmune process. Light is also used to treat babies with jaundice. But what is the evidence regarding sunlight and immune system function? There is some conflicting evidence.

For example, in a 1995 study at the University of Pennsylvania in Philadelphia, mice were inoculated with the murine (mouse) leukemia virus and exposed to one of several different lighting conditions. In one group, the mice were exposed to a constant schedule of 10 hours of light (10L) followed by 14 hours of darkness (14D). A second group was maintained in constant light (LL). A third group was exposed to a rotating schedule during which a 10L, 14D schedule was shifted every 3 days. The authors measured the amount of provirus DNA, an indicator of the amount of viral infection. They found that a week after inoculation, mice in the constant light and rotating light schedule groups had less proviral DNA than controls. Further, at 15 weeks, thymuses from control animals were showing signs of infection, while thymuses from the constant light and rotating light schedules showed no infection. It is apparent that different light schedules can alter the course of an infection although why exactly this should be the case is not entirely clear. Changing the light schedule probably changes hormonal rhythms and thus the course of infection.

Imagery

Many athletes swear by the use of visual imagery as an aid to their performance. Basketball players, for example, will often visualize a free throw swishing through the net before they shoot. Golfers as well will try to visualize what they want the ball to do before they hit it. They claim that this helps their shots. (We have tried this on the golf course and found no benefit of visualization, but there probably is a skill threshold that must be reached for the technique to be effective.) What would you say if we told you that some scientists advocate the same kind of procedure for your immune system?

Try to relax and visualize your immune cells as little Pac-Men (from the popular 1980s video game). Picture the Pac-Men eating cancer cells, which you can visualize as the little blips that Pac-Man eats. Or imagine the cancer cells as ice, with your immune system as the sun melting the cancer cells away. What if we told you that these techniques might actually help your immune system work? There are a few notable proponents of this intriguing view, although the actual empirical data supporting the idea is sparse at best.

The people most associated with imagery as an adjunct to traditional cancer treatment are O. Carl Simonton, a physician who now operates the Simonton Cancer Center in Pacific Palisades, California, and Stephanie Matthews-Simonton, a clinical psychologist. Together, they pioneered the Simonton Method, a combination of relaxation and visual imagery. Their most famous book, *Getting Well Again*, describes their experience with cancer patients who adopted their technique. The book chronicles a number of patients who either recovered or survived much longer than expected.

The Simonton Method has a number of vocal proponents, most notably cancer patients and graduates of their program. The idea itself has a number of attractive features. We all want to believe that concentrating hard enough about something will make it happen, especially if it is the elimination or reduction of cancer. We can especially describe potential pathways whereby this might work. Relaxation should lessen stress, for example, and may lead to feelings of hopefulness and a decrease in helplessness. All of these things may work separately or together to improve the status of cancer patients.

So is there a problem with these imagery techniques? Simply put, yes. There are very few controlled studies looking at imagery, and the ones that exist are often combined with another manipulation like relaxation and music. Thus, the jury is still out on imagery. Is it possible that it could work (via some of the pathways that we described) to reduce or eliminate cancer? Sure, but without the empirical support, we can't say definitively. At minimum, relaxation and using visual imagery are not dangerous or untested drugs and can't do any major harm. It should *never* be used in place of traditional therapies, however.

Prayer and Religion

A number of surveys indicate that most Americans believe in a God, believe that there is a heaven and hell, and pray on a regular basis. Belief seems to be good for a sense of purpose and meaning in our lives. What if we told you that it also seems to be good for your immune system and health? There are some fascinating data out there that state that individuals who have faith and regularly attend some kind of religious service get better faster and are generally healthier than those who don't pray. Maybe Mom was right about going to church. Let us take you through a few of the studies and what they say, then examine what the data may really mean.

One study in the late 1800s was conducted by Sir Francis Galton, a first cousin of the father of evolutionary theory, Charles Darwin. Galton was an eclectic scientist, interested in a wide variety of phenomena. He was interested in intelligence and conducted a number of measurements on a variety of people in an attempt to support his belief that intelligence was largely inherited. In his book entitled *Hereditary Genius*, he argued that intelligence was inherited because many relatives of people known for their intellect were also very bright (he modestly included himself and Darwin as examples). He also invented one formula for computing correlations, a concept that we discuss throughout the book, and was curious about the efficacy of prayer. Galton analyzed a number of cases of famous people who were sick and who were either prayed for or not. His conclusion? Prayer had no effect on whether or not the person survived. He thus concluded that prayer was ineffective. A scientist to the end.

But science hasn't necessarily verified Galton's opinion, either. Modern research has uncovered some interesting relationships between religion, prayer, and health that would make Galton's soul spin. Dale Mathews, M.D., of Georgetown University School of Medicine in Washington, D.C., has documented many of these findings in his book *The Faith Factor*. There are now a number of carefully conducted studies that seem to suggest strongly that faith is a factor in health and recovery. Here is a sampling of some of them.

A 1991 study from Northern Illinois University in DeKalb examined the relationship between religiosity and a number of health-related behaviors and outcomes. The subjects were more than 1,000 college students at Northern Illinois University, the vast majority of whom were between the ages of 17 and 22, with 59 percent of the sample group being female. Two questions were asked to assess what the authors referred to as religiosity. The first question was simply, How often do you attend religious services—never, sometimes, often, or routinely? The second question was, How religious are you? The options here were "very religious," "somewhat religious," or "not religious." The subjects filled out a questionnaire that assessed wellness, which asked about things like exercise, nutrition, stress management, and social support. Further information was collected about risky behaviors like smoking, drinking, drug use, and seat belt use.

The data collected turned up some interesting correlations. Religiosity, as they measured it, was correlated with a number of health-related behaviors. High religiosity was negatively associated with both smoking and drinking. That is, participants who described themselves as religious were less likely to smoke and drink heavily than participants with low religiosity ratings. Individuals who reported high religiosity were also more likely to use seat belts and less likely to report drug use. Finally, higher religiosity was associated with greater wellness, including regular exercise and good nutrition. What this study tells us is that individuals who report being religious are more likely to practice good health behaviors. This in and of itself is not stunning news. They should therefore have stronger immune systems via indirect mechanisms.

A similar study was published in 1995 by researchers from Eastern Virginia Medical School in Norfolk. This study also found significant relationships between religiosity and overall health status in a large sample of African-Americans. Given the data presented in the previous study, this finding is perhaps not that surprising.

One area where a number of studies have been conducted examining the effects of religion and prayer is cardiac surgery. A 1998 study conducted by researchers at the University of Michigan in Ann Arbor examined 196 patients who received coronary artery bypass graft surgery at the University of Michigan Medical Center. The patients returned questionnaires to the researchers both 6 months and 1 year after their surgeries were completed. Measures were obtained regarding religious practices as well as depression, anxiety, and health status. Individuals who reported praying privately also had less general distress 1 year after their surgeries. Individuals who prayed also had less depression 1 year after surgery than those who didn't.

The authors conclude that a possible mechanism mediating the relationship between prayer and better health outcomes may be optimism. In fact, one of the study's authors was Christopher Peterson, Ph.D., of the University of Michigan, Ann Arbor, a former student of Martin Seligman, Ph.D., of the University of Pennsylvania in Philadelphia and a noted researcher on helplessness and optimism himself. As we mentioned in previous chapters, an optimistic explanatory style is itself associated with better health. People with a strong religious faith report more optimism because they believe in the efficacy of prayer.

Another possible reason for the effectiveness of prayer is that it is related to an internal locus of control, an old psychological construct that has been studied thousands of times over the past several decades. The issue at hand is whether or not you believe that events (health-related or other) are under your control. In a number of studies, an internal locus of control has been associated with better health outcomes than an external locus of control. Simply put, things are better if you think you can do something about them, which makes intuitive sense.

A 1991 study at the University of Alabama at Birmingham did not find support for this idea, however. On the day before they underwent cardiac surgery, 100 subjects filled out a questionnaire assessing both locus of control and a "helpfulness of prayer" scale developed by the study authors. The results did not indicate a relationship between locus of control and belief in the helpfulness of prayer. There were several reasons that this was probably the case. First, 70 percent of the subjects rated prayer as extremely helpful in coping, and 96 percent reported using prayer as a coping strategy. These high values, while impressive, probably precluded a relationship with locus of control because of a lack of statistical variability. In other words, individuals with both an internal and external locus of control reported that prayer was helpful in coping. A different sample with a more diverse opinion about prayer may have turned up a relationship. These individuals believed that prayer was an effective way of coping with a health-related crisis.

These are just a few studies examining the relationship between religiosity and health. We now have to make some scientific observations. It would be easy for a person of faith to look at the studies that we just described and conclude that they provide proof for the existence of God and the efficacy of prayer. The people with strong faiths tended to do better, didn't they? That is true, but are there other explanations for why they might have gotten better?

A person who believes that he will be positively influenced by prayer is much less likely to experience depression, helplessness, and hopelessness, all of which can impair the immune system. And a strong faith will engender feelings of optimism and confidence, both of which may improve immunity and recovery. Recall our finding that a pessimistic explanatory style is correlated with lower IgA levels (see chapter 2).

So, while we are not drawing any conclusions about God or faith, what we are saying is that the presence of prayer and faith will induce known psychological processes that may aid health and recovery. Given that we are scientists, we have to interpret the data via known mechanisms that may improve the immune system. But if someone wants to interpret the described findings as evidence for a Supreme Being, more power to them (pun intended).

Getting Connected . . .
with Light, Both In and Around You

There's a lot of light out there just waiting to work its way into your immune system, and it's easy to start shedding a little on your life, both literally and figuratively. All it takes is a few minutes, an open mind—and maybe some comfy walking shoes and a pair of shades.

Take a walk. What could be more exhilarating than taking a walk on a beautiful sunny day? It improves the spirit and the body. Still, caution should be exercised. Skin cancer is the most common form of cancer, and also the most preventable. So use common sense—limit your time in direct sunlight, but enjoy it!

Imagine yourself as a better person. Visualize yourself as a better lover, public speaker, dancer, whatever. There is a plethora of self-help information out there where the message is clear: If you can imagine something, you can make it happen. This advice, perhaps overly simplistic, may also apply to immune function. Sit in a quiet and comfortable chair and actively visualize your T and B cells gobbling up any bad things that might be running around in your body. Perhaps it's the relaxation, or perhaps visualizing something actually triggers the production of immune cells. Either way, it can't hurt you.

Keep your connections. How about religion? The data are pretty clear that people with faith in God who attend services regularly are happier and also recover faster from illness. The advice therefore seems pretty clear: If you have lost touch with your church, synagogue, mosque, or other place of worship, it's a good idea to try to reconnect. It may provide you with some overarching meaning in your life, improve your network of support, and help you meet other people—all good things for immunity.

Chapter 9

Pleasure: The Final Frontier

WHERE DO WE GO FROM HERE?

There are more things in heaven and earth, Horatio, than are dreamt of in your philosophy.

—William Shakespeare, in *Hamlet*

One Sunday afternoon, as I was taking a break from work, I sat down on my backyard deck and began to enjoy some Norman Mailer. Mailer, two-time Pulitzer Prize winner and world-famous tough guy, fascinates me. I consider him the king of somatic metaphor. It shows up everywhere in his writing. Anyway, I began to read a passage from his *Tough Guys Don't Dance*, published in 1984. The experience was incredible for me since I had just been writing about cancer, the immune system, and schizophrenia. And what happens? Mailer is addressing the development of cancer caused by psychological symptoms.

He writes about Dougy "Big Mac" Madden, a hulk of a retired longshoreman, describing to his son Tim how he got cancer.

"It started 45 years ago," Big Mac states, the time he was shot several times but still chased his assailant for several blocks. As he passed St. Vincent's Hospital, he decided to stop chasing and went into the hospital to be treated. Big Mac describes this incredibly sensible act as the "first trigger." Big Mac "lost his nerve," he tells his son. This "cocked the gun." But when Tim asks what the second event was, Big Mac says that the trigger simply "corroded." "Cumulative effects. Forty-five years of living with no respect for myself." Tim says, "You're crazy," recounting how he chased the culprit for six blocks with anywhere from four to six bullets in him. This is where Big Mac states, "I wish I was. Then I wouldn't have cancer. I've studied this, I tell you. There's buried statistics if you look for them. Schizophrenics only get cancer half as often as the average population. I figure it this way: Either your body goes crazy or your mind."

It's here where Mailer actually describes how events and accompanying perceptions may lead to disorder. First of all, most disorders are from multiple causes. Hence, the two triggers: one an environmental event, the other the internal psychic consequences of the event—he had no nerve. That's why he failed to catch his assailant. Chapter 2 tells us that this is an internal, stable, and global interpretation of failure. This, we know, leads to helplessness and, in a prolonged state (like 45 years), hopelessness.

Data from our study as well as others show that this state can produce deleterious effects on the immune system. In one rat study it was shown that if a male rat assumes a defeat posture (lying on his back) when confronted by a more dominant animal, his immune system suffers for a prolonged period. If he fights back (even though he loses) rather than giving up, his immune system suffers far less dramatic consequences. Such research documents the negative effects on the human immune system, our primary defense initiative against cancer. Mailer (and Big Mac) somehow knew this before anyone else did.

Choosing Your Friends:
A Personality Profile

When it comes to boosting your immunity, it's important to be around people who will foster good feelings and affect you in positive ways. Those who possess some or all of the following traits are the best people with whom to forge friendships or spend time.

◆ Be around people who are humorous. The reasons are buried in your immune system.

◆ Hang out with optimists. They'll help you attribute causality to negative events in external, unstable, specific ways, and the opposite for positive ones (internal, stable, global).

◆ Be around people who are good conversationalists as well as good listeners. They will offer advice when you disclose your feelings, and some of it might even be good. If not, at least you've vented your feelings, they'll talk while you listen, and you'll be distracted from your negative focus on things.

◆ Be around people who are active. They're likely to instigate activity in you. This is good even if it just serves to break up depression.

◆ Be around people who are not high in power motivation. They'll just be more fun because they'll simply be happy to be with you, not try to control you. This will rub off on you if you're not a complete control freak.

Looking to Big Mac's statement about schizophrenia, we see that it's not entirely far-fetched. The hypersecretion of cytokines (molecules that kick in the immune system) that often accompanies schizophrenia (and some researchers say causes it) leads to immune system activation. Although the data regarding schizophrenia and cancer aren't at all clear, it makes some intuitive sense. Perhaps an overactive immune system protects the body at the expense of the mind. Hence, this research doesn't lie far from validating Big Mac's diatribe. To return to Mailer's metaphor, events in our lives may have already cocked the trigger, but pleasure is the anticorrosive.

The Importance of Moderation

Too much of a good thing is wonderful.—Mae West

Nothing too much.—Aristotle

What a fascinating thought: the prospect of a debate between Mae West and Aristotle. But who was right? Is too much of a good thing a great thing? We're reminded of the classic *M*A*S*H* episode where Frank Burns is giving Hawkeye and Trapper John a test to see if they are alcoholics. In response to the question "Do you drink?" Hawkeye deadpans, "Only to excess." That's funny stuff, but is excess a good thing?

Aristotle gets our vote. Although it may not be terribly surprising that a couple of academic types would pick Aristotle over Mae West, the data are on his side. Even the brain and psyche agree, according to British studies at the University of Dundee and the University of Reading. In the first study, individuals were given free access to bread and butter or chocolate (an opioid peptide agonist, or pleasure inducer) over a 22-day period. Measures were taken every 4 days through the eating period that assessed both the pleasure involved in the taste and the desire to consume the substance. The results indicated that no change of these dimensions (pleasure and desire) occurred for the palatable but non-endorphin-eliciting staples, bread and butter. At the same time, both the rated pleasurability and desire to consume chocolate plummeted over time. What does that mean? Too much of a good thing and you get sick of it. We all know this already. Picture your favorite food (maybe it is chocolate). Now picture eating that and nothing else for a few weeks straight. We're pretty sure that after a while, eating that food would be the last thing you wanted to do.

In the study at the University of Reading, done with rats, molecular biological techniques were used to ascertain exactly what happens in areas of the brain as a result of consumption of sweet substances. The results supported our position; repeated exposure to these rat delectables increased opioid peptide production, but too much of this good thing shut down receptors in the brain for these pleasure-inducing peptides.

Exercise

We are pretty much constantly bombarded with advice to get out and exercise. Run, play sports, walk—do *something*, the advice goes. Many of us listen to the advice. We head over to the gym during lunch hour or after work, change into old T-shirts, and try to get a sweat going for a period of time. People who exercise regularly report that they drop some weight, feel better about themselves, and even miss exercising if they have to skip a day or two. The literature pertaining to exercise and immune function is extraordinarily complex, but it seems generally to fit nicely in with our overarching theme: Moderation may be the key to success.

There is a scientific field called exercise immunology that examines the effect of exercise on immunological parameters. There are several findings that appear pretty consistently in this very complex literature. There is evidence, for example, that heavy or exhausting exercise may be immunosuppressive and related to increases in upper-respiratory infections. The data pertaining to more moderate bouts of exercise, relevant to the vast majority of us, are less clear. There are some reports that moderate exercise has immunoenhancing effects, but the results are not entirely consistent. Other studies report no relationship between exercise and immunity.

A number of studies have looked at the immunological effects of moderate exercise, with the aforementioned conflicting results. A 1998 study from the University of Colorado in Boulder examined the effects of a moderate bout of exercise on both young (average age of 26) and older (average age of 69) adults. Subjects were tested at rest and immediately after a 20-minute session on a treadmill at submaximal intensity. They found that lymphocyte proliferation in response to a mitogen increased by 55 percent after exercise in the young subjects. (Lymphocytes, you'll remember, are cells that play a role in detecting and destroying invaders.) Further, exercise increased the number of T lymphocytes, or T cells, in the young subjects. In the older subjects, the baseline levels of T cells were lower than in the younger subjects. Lymphocyte proliferation increased by 18 percent in the older subjects after exercise, although this increase did not reach statistical significance. The increase in T cells was comparable in the older subjects as it was in the younger subjects. The study authors concluded that although the baseline measures were lower in older subjects, they still proved the positive effects of one session of moderate exercise.

Another study examining the effect of exercise on immunity with older subjects was conducted at the University of Illinois in Chicago and published in 1999. This study differed from the previous one in that it examined the effects of 6 months of exercise as opposed to one 20-minute session. Twenty-nine older subjects (average age of 65) were assigned to either a three-times-a-week moderate exercise condition, or to a control condition that consisted of flexibility and toning training. The results indicated that some moderate gains in immune function were attained. For example, there was a trend toward an increase in T cells, but this appeared in both groups. The T cell proliferative response to a mitogen was greater in the exercise group. Finally, the activity of natural killer cells was greater in the exercise group than the control group. The changes observed in immune parameters were less than in the study above, but some increases in immune function were still observed. The differences in the two studies illustrate a general problem with assessing the effect of exercise on immunity. The type, intensity, and duration of the exercise studied all appear to be relevant. Further, the staggering number of possible immune parameters to measure further complicates the issue. In short, it will be many years before definitive answers are found to what exactly the effect is of a bout of moderate exercise.

As we mentioned, a significant amount of research has focused on intense or exhausting exercise. The data here imply that very intense exercise seems to be immunosuppressive. For example, salivary immunoglobulin A (IgA) and IgM both decline immediately after a bout of intense exercise but usually recover within 24 hours. Constant training at intense levels should cause a chronic suppression of mucosal immunity and thus an increased risk for upper respiratory tract infections. A series of studies from Australia has looked at the effect of intensive exercise in elite swimmers during training. This group has consistently found lower levels of serum IgG in the athletes compared with controls. Further, swimmers with lower levels of IgA before training were more likely to contract an upper respiratory tract infection during the 7-month training period. In a separate study, swimmers who were sick had a sharper decline in salivary IgM after a single training session than swimmers who were not ill. Finally, although the athletes seem immunosuppressed, they were able to mount responses to an oral vaccine, indicating that the immunosuppression was not global in nature.

What does all this mean? Not much to the vast majority of us, whose exercise programs are nowhere near exhaustive or elite. For elite athletes, it appears that intense exercise is immunosuppressive and may lead to more illnesses, at least for a subset of them. Although the data are pretty clear that intense exercise is a stressor that may deleteriously affect the innate immune system, the acquired-immune system appears mostly unaffected. Further, reports of increases in illness in elite athletes are not uniform. Therefore, the exercise data as a whole do not appear to get us off the hook; we should not avoid exercise because of fear of infection. The data still say that the known pluses of exercise outweigh by a mile any possible minuses.

Conditioning Your Immune System

Let's do a little free association here. Don't read ahead; just imme-diately blurt out loud the first thing that comes to mind when you read this next word: Salt.

We bet you said "Pepper." The overwhelming percentage of people will say the same thing for three reasons (commonly known as Aristotle's three laws of association): similarity, contiguity (things that occur together), and contrast. Actually, salt and pepper relate to all three. But what is of most interest to us—and to the field of psychoneuroimmunology—is the law of contiguity, because what it states is that for two things to become associated, all that needs to happen is for them to occur together. There need be no other log-ical connection between the two.

This concept is the basis of Pavlovian conditioning, as we'll de-scribe momentarily. More important, it lays the foundation for ex-citing possibilities when it comes to our immune system. It shows that by making the Immunity-Pleasure Connection in our lives, we can do more than live pleasurably, cross our fingers, and hope for good health; we can actually condition, or train, our immune sys-tems to be stronger, more efficient, and more responsive.

Saved by the Bell

Classical or Pavlovian conditioning is a simple kind of learning that was discovered by the Russian physiologist Ivan Pavlov. Pavlov was a Nobel Prize–winning physiologist interested in digestion. His early work had to do with studying the stomach secretions of dogs in re-sponse to food. Pavlov would surgically implant a tube that collected the stomach secretions of the dogs when they ate something. He then chemically analyzed the secretions. Once he had the informa-tion he thought that he needed, he logically moved up the path of digestion to the mouth, where digestion of food really begins. We all salivate in response to food; it is a reflex that we're born with. If you put some food in your mouth and leave it there, it will start to get soft and dissolve due to the presence of digestive enzymes in saliva. These enzymes were what Pavlov wished to study.

Pavlov was very careful about conducting his studies. More specifically, he fed the animals at the same time every day, fed them the same type of food, and so on. What happened after a few days both surprised and baffled him. The mere sight of the laboratory workers—even the sound of their footsteps in the hall—would cause the animals to begin salivating. This was very annoying to Pavlov because it essentially ruined his experiment. He was trying to study salivation in response to food consumption, and the dogs were salivating before food was anywhere near them.

Throughout the history of science, many important discoveries have been made as a result of experiments that have gone differently than expected. Things don't always go as expected for scientists, but great ones recognize the opportunity when something unexpected happens. This is what Pavlov did. He realized that it was extremely interesting that the animals were salivating to some mental idea related to food, and he had the courage to change his entire laboratory around to study what he called psychic secretions.

Pavlov reasoned that the cues that occurred prior to the food's presentation were signaling the dogs that food was about to be presented, thus eliciting salivation. Given this reasoning, Pavlov designed his famous experiment, and thus classical, or Pavlovian, conditioning was born. He presented a bell, which served as the cue, immediately before the food was presented to the animals. After several pairings of bell and food, voilà! Ringing of the bell alone was sufficient to elicit salivation in the animals.

Pavlov coined a number of terms as a result of his experiments. The food, as the stimulus that naturally caused a response, was the unconditioned stimulus (US). Salivation, which is the reflexive response that the US causes, was the unconditioned response (UR). The bell, an initially neutral stimulus that eventually became meaningful by being paired with the US, was the conditioned stimulus (CS). Finally, the response to the CS was the conditioned response, or CR.

Another Happy "Accident"

As with the case of Pavlov, a more recent occurrence of contiguity occurred in the laboratory of Robert Ader, Ph.D., a psychologist at the University of Rochester in New York. The resulting study, published in 1975 by Ader and his colleague, immunologist Nathan Cohen, Ph.D., described actual conditioning of the immune system. This study really began psychoneuroimmunology (PNI) in many ways and has led to a significant amount of research.

Dr. Ader was actually attempting to study taste aversion learning, a special variant of classical conditioning with which you're probably familiar. A taste aversion develops when you experience a particular taste, then become ill. Whether or not the item you ate was what actually made you ill is beside the point; you still develop an aversion to that taste. Most of us have at least one food to which we have an aversion, and the phenomenon has clear biological relevance. Animals in the wild that eat something and then become ill will tend to stop eating what they believe made them ill.

Dr. Ader was a learning psychologist and was interested in taste aversion learning for several esoteric reasons that we won't bore you with. He was studying mice and presenting them with a novel taste, saccharin, as the CS (conditioned stimulus). Rodents have a sweet tooth like humans, and will readily eat or drink sweet substances. As for the US (unconditioned stimulus), which was supposed to produce nausea, they used the drug cyclophosphamide. Dr. Ader and Dr. Cohen were attempting to extinguish the aversion to the saccharin by presenting it repeatedly by itself. (This is how you eliminate or extinguish a classically conditioned response: by presenting the CS alone a number of times.) A significant number of the mice, when presented with the saccharin a number of times, got sick. Some of them even died.

Preparing for Oncology Clinic Visits

While cancer clinics do not occasion a celebratory mood, why not do all that's possible to make a bad situation more bearable? Even if we can't elicit major pleasurable sensations, maybe we can at least buffer stress during the several-hour visit with the following recommendations.

1. Predominant colors should be pastels (see "Kicks for Kids" on page 182).

2. Lighting should be lower intensity, broad spectrum radiation (see chapter 8).

3. Loud equipment "beeps" and the like should be piped into an enclosed nurse's station (see chapter 4).

4. Headphones and tape decks should play 30 minutes of favorite music (see chapter 4).

5. Headphones, VCR, and color monitors should provide 30 minutes of a favorite situation comedy (see chapter 7).

6. About 20 minutes should be spent consuming a favorite meal with an accompanying chocolate dessert (remember to sniff the chocolate; see chapter 9).

7. Every 10 minutes, someone should prompt five very deep breaths (see chapter 3).

8. A pen and paper with hours of the day printed on it should allow for at least 15 minutes of planning an entire forthcoming Saturday of pleasurable events, including detailed meals and activities (see "13-Point Pleasure Formula" on page 181).

9. Intermittent time should be spent throughout the visit conversing and holding hands with a favorite person (see chapter 5).

10. And just for the heck of it, at least 10 minutes should be spent imagining the chemotherapeutic infusion drowning the cancer cells in the bloodstream (see chapter 8).

11. A 20-minute snooze couldn't hurt either (see chapter 1).

While these recommendations certainly won't cure cancer, research tells us that they may very well help. At worst, this several-hour visit will become much more tolerable under these circumstances. And while you can't paint the clinic walls for yourself or your loved one, you can make a tape and bring a portable headset. So exert as much control over the situation as you can. This alone will pay psychological and immune-system dividends.

The researchers thought that the result was a little odd, until they recognized that cyclophosphamide, the drug that they had used to induce nausea, was also an immunosuppressant agent. Since the saccharin had been paired with the drug, they thought that maybe what they were observing was a conditioned immunosuppression. If a completely innocent taste could produce illness simply by being paired with an immunosuppressive drug, why couldn't a taste also produce the immunosuppressive effects? They thus designed the seminal experiment that really began psychoneuroimmunology as a discipline.

Here's the experiment that they performed. Mice were again exposed to a novel taste, saccharin, as they were exposed to the cyclophosphamide. The mice were also injected with the red blood cells of sheep, which should initiate the formation of antibodies. The taste served as the CS, while the drug was the US, the stimulus that automatically causes an effect. What they found was really astonishing, especially for the time. Mice that were exposed to the taste and drug together, and then reexposed to the CS (taste), showed lower antibody levels against the red blood cells than mice that were not reexposed to the saccharin CS, or that were exposed to the saccharin but never had it paired with the cyclophosphamide. Dr. Ader and Dr. Cohen ran all of the appropriate control groups, and the result was clear: Saccharin by itself does not produce immunosuppression, but it will if it is paired with an immunosuppressive drug. The immune system can be conditioned.

As we mentioned, this astonishing finding really began PNI. Prior to this study, we were already aware of a number of things that could suppress immunity as part of their inherent activity. We now know from this research, however, that neutral events can become immunosuppressive if they happen to be paired with immunosuppressive agents or events. The fact that immune system function could be conditioned was groundbreaking. This basic phenomenon has been replicated a number of times in a number of species. Other immunosuppressive agents, such as morphine, can serve as the US and thus support conditioning. Conditioned immunosuppression has been demonstrated in rats, mice, and humans. Moreover, T lymphocyte (T cell) as well as B lymphocyte (B cell) antibodies have been shown to respond to conditioning. Even nonspecific immune responses, such as complement and lysozymes, are subject to conditioning. This is a widespread phenomenon.

Dr. Ader and Dr. Cohen did some astonishing follow-up experiments exploring some of the implications of their findings. They asked a simple question: When would it be a good thing to suppress the immune system? They had an answer, described in one of the follow-up studies published in 1982. This experiment utilized a strain of mice genetically susceptible to lupus erythematosus, an autoimmune disease. Humans with autoimmune diseases such as lupus are often given immunosuppressive drugs as part of their treatment. Since their immune systems are attacking themselves, the drugs are used to reduce symptoms. Immunosuppressive drugs are pretty nasty, however, producing lots of side effects. Therefore, if it were possible to somehow slow down the immune system without producing all of the nasty side effects, you would have a very effective treatment. But how could you do that?

In this study, cyclophosphamide was again paired with saccharine. Ordinarily, the immunosuppressive drug must be given weekly to delay symptoms. If it is given every other week, no positive benefits are accrued. In this study, however, after the saccharin taste was paired with the drug, saccharin administered alone every other week was sufficient to slow the development of symptoms. There was also a decrease in mortality. This is a very desirable effect—the reduction of disease symptoms with half of the nasty drug. Animals that received saccharin without cyclophosphamide did not show the same effect, nor did animals that received both saccharin and the drug, but not in combination.

Would this kind of thing work in humans? Dr. Ader addressed

this critical question in a 1992 study. The methodology was essentially the same as the one we just described, except that instead of mice, the subject was an 11-year-old girl suffering from severe lupus. The normal treatment regimen for lupus would be 12 (1 per month) treatments with cyclophosphamide, the immunosuppressive agent mentioned previously. As we also mentioned, this is a nasty drug that produces lots of side effects. The girl was given six pairings of a cod-liver-oil taste and rose-perfume smell (together they were the CS) with her cyclophosphamide (US). This pairing was given to her every other month, with the combination CS given by itself every other month. The girl showed a significant reduction in symptoms during the year she was studied, as well as fewer side effects. Remember, she received only half of the usual dose of drug. Further, she was examined 5 years later and was still doing well. Obviously, a single case study does not constitute an experiment, but the results are still striking. They suggest that conditioning could be used as an effective adjunct treatment for individuals suffering from autoimmune disease.

If conditioned immunosuppression has utility for those rare individuals with autoimmune disorders, could conditioning be used to improve immune functioning? There are not many studies, but there are a few with intriguing results. Individuals with AIDS, for example, have an impaired immune system that makes them susceptible to a variety of opportunistic infections. There have been several reports of conditioned enhancement in AIDS patients. Other reports have been unable to replicate the findings. The scientific jury is still out on whether the immune system can be boosted as easily as it can be suppressed.

Although the majority of data regarding classical conditioning and immune function has focused on immune suppression, there are a number of studies that demonstrate that conditioned enhancement of immunity is also possible. For example, a research group from Germany has published a number of studies using human subjects. It is well known that an injection of epinephrine (adrenaline)

in humans will lead to an increase in both NK cell number and activity. In one study, humans were presented with a sweet taste,
which served as the CS, and then immediately given an injection of
epinephrine (US). This was done for 4 consecutive days. On day 5,
subjects were exposed to the CS by itself. The subjects showed a significant increase in NK cell activity (to a sweet taste!), as large as a
group actually given epinephrine that day. The researchers ran all of
the appropriate control groups, and the effect seems clearly due to
conditioning. This is a powerful demonstration that the immune
system can also be conditioned to work better, not just conditioned
to be inhibited.

One question that must currently go unanswered about these
kinds of findings asks whether the immune system itself gets conditioned or whether other physiological systems (epinephrine or cortisol, for example) get conditioned, thereby affecting immunity. In
other words, is it simply cortisol or some other hormone that is the
CR, and is the effect on immunity indirect? Or are immune cells
and organs themselves directly conditioned? This important question has yet to be resolved.

Pleasure and Guilt

If pleasure is the immune system's savior, then guilt is its counter-
point nemesis. A number of studies have shown a close connection
between pleasure and guilt. Guilt is that aversive set of emotional
consequences that we feel when we have committed an act that we
consider some sort of transgression, usually involving inflicting some
sort of harm upon another (but it could also be directed toward an
animal, a part of our environment, or ourselves). Guilt serves to
punish behaviors that we consider unacceptable by levying mental
torture as our sentence. It is a stress elicitor and is related to the initiation of depression.

Consider the following scenario: Margie sits at her favorite downtown restaurant one night and, after a long and ponderous debate, decides to indulge her yen for chocolate. Margie is 5 feet 7 inches tall, weighs 125 pounds, is in perfect health, and rarely allows herself such gastronomic pleasures. Here's a great, rare opportunity for some immune-boosting elicitation of opioid peptides in Margie, right? Wrong.

What she has done is set off a vicious cycle of mental torture regarding her health, her figure, and her general well-being. She is so overwhelmed with guilt that she can hardly stand it. Consequently, rather than enjoying an immune system boost from the dessert, the stress-induced effects of cortisol and the immune-system-numbing depression that sets in has such deleterious effects on her immune system that Death by Chocolate becomes her epitaph rather than the name of her favorite dessert.

This is truly a tragedy. Margie has a healthy lifestyle, and all she needs to do to help maintain it is experience some common pleasures occasionally, but the psyche of this woman just won't permit it. She turns beneficial, pleasurable activities into immune system catastrophes. How about taking a few days off from work to relax and enjoy life? Don't even go there—she'd be a basket case. But Margie isn't so unusual. An international study shows that people are the same way in Australia, Germany, Italy, Spain, Switzerland, the United Kingdom, and other Western countries.

Similarly, in another international study, 4,000 adults were surveyed regarding everyday pleasurable activities and guilt. The participants came from Australia, Belgium, Germany, Italy, the Netherlands, Spain, Switzerland, and the United Kingdom. Each individual rated 13 everyday presumably pleasurable activities on a scale of 0 to 10, where 0 indicated no enjoyment at all and 10 was extremely enjoyable. These ratings were analyzed in concert with whether they also sometimes or often felt guilty about enjoying the particular object or activity. An extremely important, though not surprising, finding from an immune system perspective was that as guilt went up, pleasure went down. This inverse relationship between guilt and pleasure showed sexual activity and listening to

---

13-Point Pleasure Formula

Take an evening to try this easy formula for getting pleasure into your life, and see just how wonderful boosting your immunity can be.

1. Sniff and eat a piece of chocolate (see "Pleasure and Guilt" on page 179). Dark is preferable, but milk chocolate is fine. Let it melt in your mouth.

2. Pet Rover or play with Fluffy (see chapter 6).

3. Pick up the phone and make reservations at your favorite restaurant for tomorrow night with your two best friends. You get bonus points if they're upbeat people (see "Choosing Your Friends" on page 167).

4. Put on your favorite article of clothing, look in the mirror, and smile. Tell yourself you look marvelous, and remember this statement for the rest of the evening (see chapter 2).

5. Turn on the stereo and play your favorite CD (see chapter 4).

6. Pour a glass of Cabernet Sauvignon for yourself and a partner, spouse, or friend. Now sit back, relax, and talk (see chapter 2).

7. Treat yourself and your mate to reciprocal massages (see chapter 5).

8. Watch a funny movie or tune in to your favorite sitcom. Don't hesitate to laugh out loud (see chapter 7).

9. Hug, kiss, and have a sexual encounter with your mate (see chapter 5).

10. Before having sex, dim the lights in the room (see chapter 8).

11. Throughout the evening, remember to breathe slowly and deeply, and take time to enjoy the relaxing feeling (see chapter 3).

12. Vividly imagine and relive in your mind a wonderful event in your life (see chapter 8).

13. Now say your evening prayers, if you're so inclined (see chapter 8). If you're still alert and awake, plan a whole day full of pleasurable activities for the weekend (see chapter 2). Now, get a good night's sleep (see chapter 1).

---

music in the lowest-scoring guilt group. Middle-of-the-road guilt was ascribed to sports, exercise, eating at restaurants and vendors, eating dairy products, drinking tea and coffee, watching TV, and shopping for treats. At the top of the guilt induction scale was smoking, eating chocolates, and eating sweets like cake and ice cream.

Kicks for Kids:
A Pleasure Formula for Children

Nothing beats early intervention. So we've developed a downsized version of our Immunity-Pleasure Connection for baby. Below are 10 pleasurable tips for giving your infant's immune system a head start.

Breastfeed your newborn. It's nutritionally sound, and it's a great way for Mommy to bond with baby. Also, baby receives the positive stimulus of being touched by Mom, which is great for the immune system. And the big bonus is that colostrum (breast milk during the first couple of weeks) is loaded with immunoglobulin A (IgA).

Play music. Do this prenatally and neonatally, and continue postnatally into childhood. Studies have shown that babies in utero respond to this. The music affects their heart rate and oxygen saturation.

Make baby laugh by tickling him gently.

Please baby's visual sense with color. Pastels are calming and peaceful, which is great for the immune system. But primary colors stimulate pleasure, also great for the immune system. The solution is to have long periods of peace and relaxation interspersed frequently with pleasure, so paint the nursery walls a pale pastel color and entertain baby with red toys like balls.

Make Mom's presence known. Babies love to feel Mommy's touch, and

Interestingly, the Dutch, as compared with all other groups, avoided the guilt trap. They tended to relax and enjoy their everyday pleasures. The Germans were very uptight, and the British were second in mastery of the hedonic, but they also pay for it with guilt more than the average person afterward. The Italians felt most deprived by their guilt, and one-third of the entire sample said that they'll just carry it with them as part of their lives.

Not included in the international studies, the French and Americans were, however, included in a study co-authored by Paul Rozin, Ph.D., a psychologist at the University of Pennsylvania in Philadelphia. First of all, let's consider the French paradox. We know that the they become fascinated with seeing her face, particularly her eyes. Studies show that at about 8 weeks after birth, opioid peptides are released in Baby by this familiarity. (By the way, seeing and touching Dad will have similar effects on Baby.)

Show Junior how to pet the dog. Engaging in behavior directed toward the dog will produce reciprocal responses. This will build the realization that his (positive) responses will be followed by (positive) outcomes in his environment.

Play peek-a-boo. This almost always makes children laugh. After hiding for the fifth time, wait for a verbal utterance, then appear to say "Boo!" Continue this, and your child will think that he's producing your appearance. (Control at a very early age helps children feel pleasure.)

Be predictable. If a babysitter is coming over, wave bye-bye to your child so that she knows you're leaving the house. She won't like that you're leaving, but her T cells will thank you.

Kids love praise. A smile and a positive comment can elicit enormous pleasure.

Try some chocolate. Studies show that chocolate in moderation has positive effects on the immune system. So cuddle up on the couch with your child and pop a few chocolates.

French rank right up there among the people with the worst diets in the world. Anything considered good in France is loaded with fat. Yet even with their fat consumption, the French experience lower incidence of heart disease, it is thought by way of wine flavonoids. While this is true, let's take another look at how the French eat as compared, for example, with Americans. Incidentally, more than 30 percent of Americans are overweight enough to be labeled obese, while less than 8 percent of the fat-consuming French are in the same category. So we learn from this that you are not necessarily what you eat.

The red-wine-and-exercise explanations of this French paradox have given way to another that fits very nicely with what we have been talking about. When Dr. Rozin compared the attitudes of both cultures, he found that the French savor the taste of their food—eating is a pleasurable experience to be engaged with nothing but enjoyment—while for the American counterparts, "every bite is both a pleasure in the mouth and a worry about what's going to happen when it gets into the body." He states that "we're getting fatter as we worry about getting fat." The French are not as worried about getting fat, and they're not getting fatter."

The question is, Can we figure out how to rid the Americans of their guilt, their concern, and their anxiety toward food? The lyrics of the old popular French song resound here: "to regret nothing . . . in matters of love and food." So don't let guilt buffer any of your pleasure. If it doesn't hurt anyone and it feels good, just do it, and enjoy every second—your immune system will.

Don't take this advice lightly. A 1999 study conducted by professionals in the department of psychology at the School of Nursing and Medical Research Laboratory at the University of Hull in England required participants to list their pleasurable activities and rate them in terms of pleasure and guilt. Afterward, they collected saliva samples and assayed them for immunoglobulin A (IgA) concentrations. Results showed a significant positive correlation between the number of pleasures and IgA specifically in women, and a significant negative correlation between guilt and IgA. The data also revealed a significant positive correlation between IgA levels and a pleasure/guilt ratio, indicating that guilt will in fact buffer the immune-system-boosting properties of pleasure when measured as a function of overall quantity of pleasure to guilt in one's life.

Final Thoughts

Some people may make the common mistake of overinterpreting the Immunity-Pleasure Connection. Are we saying that you should listen to some music, get a dog, or rent a funny video and you'll never get sick? Of course not. Someone could do every single thing that we have suggested throughout the entire book and still get a cold or still get cancer. We are not saying that pleasurable behaviors are the only influences on the immune system. What we are saying is that pleasurable activities can positively influence the immune system.

We envision health or sickness as the end products of an exceedingly complex equation, many of the variables still unknown. Your genes, that wonderful set of instructions supplied by your parents that produced you, is unquestionably relevant for your health. You can't control your eye color, your hair color, and a portion of your personality. Despite what some people may tell you, genes matter. As an example, if you are one of those rare individuals born with a congenital immune defect, music or pets won't cure you. For the rest of us, enviormental influences can make a difference.

Let's say that your overall health is 50 percent a result of your genetic background. That might sound pretty depressing. However, what that means is that 50 percent is not. We all accept this already with things like heart disease and cancer. If you smoke, your risk for both of these goes up dramatically. If you eat poorly and don't exercise, your risk increases further. If you drink excessively for years, you will probably get liver disease. Everyone already accepts that behavior is extremely relevant for health; we are just taking things a little farther. Maybe behavior and personality are more relevant for health than we ever imagined.

Behaviors that are pleasurable, as a rule, tend to be associated with boosts in immune function, as measured by a variety of techniques. Some of the boosts are quite modest, but they can add up. Small increases in immune function from several sources might together add up to a large boost. This may tip that complex equation so you don't get sick.

We must exercise caution. Plenty of folks will be happy to rub magnets on your head to "heal" you if you pay them to, but that doesn't mean that it will work. We have steadfastly covered only scientific studies. As unusual as some of them we described were, they were, in fact, studies. If they had obvious weaknesses, we tried to

A Noseful of Immune Benefits

If eating chocolate elicits too much guilt to buffer your stress and keep your immunoglobulin A levels up, the British have a solution: Just sniff it. The results of a study were presented at the British Psychophysiology Society Meeting in London in 1998, and they addressed immune system function in reaction to olfactory stimuli (smells). The researchers from the Psychophysiology and Stress Research Group at the University of Westminster placed individuals in a situation involving blindfolding, which was shown to have negative effects on IgA in the control group. Two experimental groups in addition were exposed to the smell of rotting meat and the smell of freshly melted chocolate.

The researchers reported that while sniffing the rotten meat produced a substantial decline in IgA, the pleasurable effects of sniffing chocolate buffered the negative effects of the situation as a whole (lessening the decline of IgA), while sniffing the rotten meat produced the ill effects. An interesting aside in this research shows that in a subjective evaluation of the two smells, females' ratings indicated stark differences between the effects of the rotting meat and the more calming effect of chocolate, while males' responses were more subdued. Yet, at the same time, the males exhibited more substantial immune system changes than the females. Go figure—maybe males are just more walk than talk.

point them out. In some instances we have speculated beyond what the data say. But we hope that the data indicate a clear trend.

Let's assume for a second that everything we told you is wrong. Let's say that 100 new studies are done and show that music has no effect on IgA; that social support is irrelevant for surviving an illness; that laughter does nothing for NK cells; that petting a dog is not helpful; and so on. First, we'd be very surprised. Second, remember our advice to you throughout the book: Try to develop a network of close friends and family you can rely on. Get a cat or a dog and spoil him with love. Listen to some relaxing music. Try to reduce your stress level. Be optimistic. Laugh and it will do no harm.

Glossary

acquired immunity: an immune system response that involves prior exposure to a specific antigen that creates memory for that antigen and the subsequent ability to produce antibodies against it quickly

acquired immunodeficiency syndrome (AIDS): a disease caused by the HIV retrovirus that destroys helper T cells and thus makes one susceptible to a variety of opportunistic diseases (e.g., cancer, pneumonia)

anhedonia: inability to experience pleasure

antibody: a protein produced by B lymphocytes that recognizes and acts to rid the body of antigens

antigen: any foreign substance in the body that is capable of producing an immune system response (*anti*body *gen*erator)

attributional style questionnaire (ASQ): questionnaire designed to measure your explanatory style, or way of explaining events

autonomic nervous system: the automatic part of the peripheral nervous system that is involved in such response systems as stress and emotions

B cell: lymphocytes that mature in bone marrow and transform into plasma cells that secrete antibodies

basophil: a cell involved in allergic reactions

catecholamines: hormones like epinephrine and norepinephrine that are released by the sympathetic nervous system as an immediate response to stress, initiating the fight-or-flight response

CD4 cell: a subset of T cells that includes helper T cells and inflammatory T cells that are responsible for signaling B cells to produce antibodies and bring phagocytes to a wound or laceration

CD8 cell: a subset of T cells that includes cytoxic T cells and suppressor T cells that are responsible for killing antigen and suppressing immune response (important in autoimmune disorders)

cell-mediated immunity: an immune system response initiated by B lymphocytes and T lymphocytes directed against bacteria, viruses, and cancer

central nervous system: the brain and spinal cord

cognitive dissonance: a dissociation between belief and reality that produces discomfort

complement: a system of serum proteins capable of rupturing the cell membrane

concanavalin A: a mitogen that is extracted from jack beans that causes T cell proliferation

conditioned response (CR): a positively or negatively valanced response to a conditioned stimulus (CS)

conditioned stimulus (CS): a previously neutral stimulus that has taken on the ability to elicit a positive or negative response due to association with an unconditioned stimulus (US)

cortisol: a hormone secreted by the adrenal glands during stress that can suppress immune system function

cytokine: a substance secreted by nervous or immune system cells that communicates between and within these systems and typically produces immune system activation

cytolytic: the ability to kill cells by rupturing the cell membrane

cytotoxic: the ability to kill cells

dynorphin: an opioid substance whose release in the central nervous system is correlated with both reduced pain and the initiation of pleasure

endogenous opiates: naturally occurring substances in the body, such as endorphin and enkephalin, that produce effects similar to opiates like morphine

endorphin: an opioid substance whose release in the central system is correlated with both reduced pain and the initiation of pleasure

enkephalin: an opioid substance whose release in the central nervous system is correlated with both reduced pain and the initiation of pleasure

eosinophil: a cell involved in allergic reactions and protection from parasites

Epstein-Barr virus: a virus that once contracted remains latent in an individual, and whose subsequent activation can lead to a lymphoma, infectious mononucleosis, or chronic fatigue syndrome

explanatory style: your characteristic way of explaining why events happen to you

glucocorticoids: hormones such as cortisol, produced by the adrenal gland in times of stress, that increase blood sugar

helper T cell: a subset of T cells responsible for signaling B cells to secrete antibodies in the presence of an antigen

HIV (human immunodeficiency virus): a virus that infects CD4 T cells and causes AIDS

human leukocyte group A (HLA): the major histocompatibility complex in humans

humoral immunity: the branch of the immune system responsible for immunoglobulin production, whose job it is to prevent and eliminate antigenic presence in combination with other immune system components

immune system: a complex of five major systems whose function is to prevent entrance and eliminate the presence of antigens in the bodily system

immunocompetence: one's ability to defend oneself against disease entities via the immune system

immunoenhancement: the use of various agents or sets of circumstances of a physical, psychological, or environmental nature to improve some aspect of immune system function

immunoglobulin: an antibody

immunoglobulin A (IgA): the most prevalent of the major systemic antibodies, whose function it is to prevent antigenic entry to the body and to interact with other immune system components to destroy existing antigens in the body

immunoglobulin D (IgD): one of the five major systemic antibodies, whose function is largely unknown at this time

immunoglobulin E (IgE): a major antibody whose function is largely confined to allergic reactions and defense against parasites

immunoglobulin G (IgG): a major antibody responsible for long-term protection from infection

immunoglobulin M (IgM): a major antibody involved in short-term protection, typically at times of physical insult to the body

immunosuppression: the act of producing a decrease in function in any of the major subsystems of the immune system

inflammatory response: an influx of helper T cells and phagocytes to the site of tissue damage for protection

innate immunity: defenses that exist in the body prior to exposure to a specific antigen

interferons: a major group of cytokines involved in communication between the central nervous system and the immune system

interleukins: a major group of cytokines involved in communication between the central nervous system and the immune system (e.g., IL-1, IL-2, IL-6)

lymphatic system: a system involving the spleen and lymph nodes, responsible for filtering antigens from the body *lymphocyte:* a cell that recognizes and responds to antigens

lymphoma: a cancer that proliferates as tumors found in cells of the lymphatic system

macrophage: an immune system cell whose name means "big eater"

major histocompatibility complex (MHC): genes found in every cell, responsible for moving antigens to the cell surface

mitogen: a substance that elicits cell proliferation

monoclonal antibody: specific antibodies cloned from a single cell

monocyte: a phagocyte that circulates briefly in the bloodstream and then migrates to the tissues and becomes a macrophage

mucosal associated lymphoidal tissue (MALT): lymphoid cells in the respiratory and gastrointestinal systems

natural killer cells (NK cells): large lymphocytes that engage in cytotoxic destruction of antigens

neutrophil: a phagocyte involved in inflammatory responses and cell-mediated cytotoxic action

nonspecific effector system: free-roaming monocytes, neutrophils, macrophages, and natural killer cells capable of engaging in phagocytosis and cytotoxic action

optimism: making external, unstable, and specific explanations for negative life events

parasympathetic nervous system: the part of the autonomic nervous system involved in relaxation and positive emotional states

pathogen: a disease-producing antigen

peripheral nervous system: the part of the nervous system that does not include the brain and spinal cord

pessimism: making internal, stable, and global explanations for negative life events

Peyer's patches: lymphoid cells in the small intestine

phagocyte: a variety of cells including monocytes, macrophages, and neutrophils that engulf and kill antigens

phytohemagglutinin: a T cell mitogen derived from kidney beans

pokeweed mitogen: a B cell mitogen derived from pokeweed

power motive: the desire to impact the environment or persuade or influence others

pro-inflammatory cytokines: IL-1, IL-6, and TNF

prostaglandin: a neuropeptide involved in such phenomena as pain production *psychoneuroimmunology (PNI):* field of psychology and medicine devoted to immune system interactions with the nervous system and psychological variables

Rahe Life Stress Scale: one of the psychological standard tests for assessing stress

reticuloendothelial system (RES): phagocytes found in connective tissue throughout the body

retrovirus: an RNA virus that uses reverse transcriptase to reproduce

rheumatoid factor: an auto antibody found in individuals with rheumatoid arthritis or a variety of connective tissue disorders

seasonal affective disorder (SAD): a kind of depression initiated by inadequate exposure to sunlight

self-esteem: subjective feelings of competency or worth

stable dimension: tendency to allow the repercussions of incidents to linger in the mind

stress: a reaction in the body to a perceived threat, either real or imagined, physical or psychological, that we're not certain we can handle successfully

suppressor T cells: a subset of T cells whose job it is to stop cytotoxic action, i.e., inhibit autoimmune responses

sympathetic nervous system: the branch of the autonomic nervous system involved in stress, anxiety, emergency situations, and negative emotional states

T cell: lymphocytes that mature and differentiate in the thymus

thymus: an organ found behind the breastbone where T cells mature and differentiate

transforming growth factor (TGF): a cytokine involved in multiple functions, including limiting inflammatory response and promoting wound healing

tumor necrosis factor (TNF): a cytokine that initiates inflammatory responses and destroys tumors

vaccination: introduction of a relatively harmless version of a pathogen to stimulate the production of antibodies to protect against further exposure

unconditioned response (UR): a positive or negative response automatically elicited by an unconditioned stimulus (US)

unconditioned stimulus (US): any stimulus that naturally, automatically, reliably elicits a positive or negative response

unstable dimension: tendency to view the repercussions of incidents as temporary

virulence: the strength or infectious potency of a pathogen

References

Introduction

Benedetti, F., and Amanzio, M. (1997). The neurobiology of placebo analgesia: From endogenous opioids to cholecystokinin. *Progress in Neurobiology* 51, 109–125.

Blalock, J. E. (1984). The immune system as a sensory organ. *Journal of Immunology* 132, 1067–1070.

Buckalew, L. W., and Coffield, K. E. (1982). An investigation of drug expectancy as a function of capsule color and size preparation form. *Journal of Clinical Psychopharmacology* 2, 245–248.

Crick, F. *The Astonishing Hypothesis*. New York: Touchstone Books, 1995.

Evans, F. J. Expectancy, therapeutic instructions and the placebo response. *Placebo: Theory, Research, and Mechanisms*, 215–228; eds. L. White, B. Tursky, and G. E. Schwartz. New York: Guilford, 1985.

Hawkes, C. H. (1992). Endorphins: The basis of pleasure? *Journal of Neurology, Neurosurgery and Psychiatry* 55 (4), 247–250.

Lehrman, N. S. (1993). Pleasure heals. *Archives of Internal Medicine* 153, 929–934.

Morgan, L. G. (1998). Psychoneuroimmunology, the placebo effect and chiropractic. *Journal of Manipulative and Physiological Therapeutics* 21 (7), 484–491.

Salzet, M.; Didier, V.; and Day, R. (2000). Crosstalk between nervous and immune systems through the animal kingdom: Focus on opioids. *Trends in Neurosciences* 23 (11), 550–555.

Stefano, G. B., et al. (2001). The placebo effect and relaxation response: neural processes and their coupling to constitutive nitric oxide. *Brain Research Reviews* 35, 1–19.

Van Epps, D. E., and Saland, L. (1984). Beta-endorphin and metenkephalin stimulate human peripheral blood mononuclear cell chemotaxin. *Journal of Immunology* 132, 3046–3053.

Wall, P. D. Pain and the placebo response. *Experimental and Theoretical Studies of Consciousness*, 187–216; Ciba Foundation Symposium, 174. New York: Wiley, 1993.

Chapter 1

Abbas, A. K.; Lichtman, A. H.; and Pober, J. S. *Cellular and Molecular Immunology*. Philadelphia: W. B. Saunders, 1994.

Abdou, N. I.; Pascual, E.; and Racela, L. S. (1979). Supressor T-cell function and anti-suppressor antibody in active early arthritis. *Arthritis and Rheumatism* 22, 586.

Allardyce, R. A., and Bienenstock, J. (1984). The mucosal immune system in health and disease, with an emphasis on parasitic infection. *Bulletin of the World Health Organization* 62, 7.

Antoni, M. H. (1987). Neuroendocrine influences in psychoimmunology and neoplasia: A review. *Psychology and Health* 1, 3–24.

Cancer Facts and Figures (1995). Atlanta: American Cancer Society, Inc.

Fischer, A., and Konig, W. (1991). Influence of cytokines and cellular interactions on the glucocorticoid-induced Ig (E, G, A, M) synthesis of peripheral blood mononuclear cells. *Immunology* 74, 228–233.

Foley, F. W., et al. (1988). Psychoimmunological dysregulation in multiple sclerosis. *Psychosomatics* 29, 398–403.

Kuby, J. *Immunology*. New York: W. H. Freeman and Co., 1992.

Maier, S. F., and Watkins, L. R. (1999). Bidirectional communication between the brain and the immune system: Implications for behavior. *Animal Behavior* 57 (4), 741–751.

Muller, N., and Acken, N. (1998). Psychoneuroimmunology and the cytokine action in the CNS: Implications for psychiatric disorders. *Progress in Neuro-Psychopharmacology and Biological Psychiatry* 22, 1–33.

Ogra, P. L. (1985). Local immune responses. *British Medical Bulletin* 41, 28.

Penicoff, K. D., et al. (1987). The neuropsychiatric effects of treatment with interleukin-2 and lymphokine-activated killer cells. *Annals of Internal Medicine* 107, 293–300.

Rogers, M. P., and Fordar, M. (1996). Psychoneuroimmunology of autoimmune disorders. *Advances in Neuroimmunology* 6, 169–177.

Roitt, I. M.; Brostaff, J.; and Male, D. K. *Immunology*. Philadelphia: J. B. Lippincott Co., 1989.

Rossen, R. D., et al. (1970). The protein in nasal secretions. *Journal of the American Medical Association* 211, 1157–1161.

Tomassi, T. B. *The Immune System of Secretions*. Englewood Cliffs, NJ: Prentice-Hall, 1976.

Underdown, B. J., and Schiff, J. M. (1986). Immunoglobulin A: Strategic defense initiative at the mucosal surface. *Annual Review of Immunology* 4, 389–417.

Yodfat, Y., and Silvian, H. (1977). A prospective study of acute respiratory infections among children in a kibbutz. *Journal of Infectious Disease* 135, 26–30.

Young, L. D. (1992). Psychological factors in rheumatoid arthritis. *Journal of Consulting and Clinical Psychology* 60, 619–627.

Chapter 2

Arnetz, B. B., et al. (1987). Immune function in unemployed women. *Psychosomatic Medicine* 49, 3–12.

Baggish, J. *How Your Immune System Works*. Emeryville, CA: Ziff Davis, 1994.

Bovbjerg, D. H., and Valdimarsdottir, H. (1993). Familial cancer, emotional distress, and low natural cytotoxic activity in healthy women. *Annals of Oncology* 4, 743–752.

Brennan, F. X., and Charnetski, C. J. (2000). Explanatory style and immunoglobulin A (IgA). *Integrative Physiological and Behavioral Science* 35, 251–255.

Burger, R. A., and Warren, R. P. (1998). Possible immunogenetic basis for autism. *Mental Retardation and Developmental Disabilities Research Reviews* 4, 137–141.

Connor, T. J., and Leonard, B. E. (1998). Depression, stress and immunological activation: The role of cytokines in depressive disorders. *Life Sciences* 62 (7), 583–606.

Dattore, P. J.; Shanta, F. C.; and Coyne, L. (1980). Premorbid personality differentiation of cancer and non-cancer groups: A test of the hypothesis of cancer proneness. *Journal of Consulting and Clinical Psychology* 48, 388–394.

Dean, C., and Surtees, P.G. (1989). Do psychological factors predict survival in breast cancer? *Journal of Psychosomatic Research* 33, 561–569.

Derogatis, L. R.; Abeloff, M. D.; and Melisaratos, N. (1979). Psychological coping mechanisms and survival time in metastatic breast cancer. *Journal of the American Medical Association* 242, 1504–1508.

Esterling, B. A., et al. (1994). Emotional disclosure through writing or speaking modulates latent Epstein-Barr virus antibody titers. *Journal of Consulting and Clinical Psychology* 62, 130–140.

Esterling, B. A., et al. (1993). Emotional repression, stress disclosure responses, and Epstein-Barr viral capsid antigen titers. *Psychosomatic Medicine* 52, 397–410.

Fawzy, F. I., et al. (1993). Malignant melanoma: effects of an early structured psychiatric intervention, coping and affective state on recurrence and survival 6 years later. *Archives of General Psychology* 50, 681–689.

Fife, A.; Beasley, P. J.; and Fertig, D. L. (1996). Psychoneuroimmunology and cancer: Historical perspectives and current research. *Advances in Neuroimmunology* 6, 179–190.

Futterman, P. H., et al. (1994). Immunological variability associated with experimentally induced positive and negative affective states. *Psychosomatic Medicine* 22, 231–268.

Futterman, P. H., et al. (1992). Short-term immunological effects of induced emotion. *Psychosomatic Medicine* 54, 133–148.

Gavrilova, E. A., and Shabanova, L. F. (1998). Stress-induced disorders of immune function and their psychocorrection. *Human Physiology* 24 (1), 114–121.

Greer, S.; Morris, T.; and Pettingale, K. W. (1979). Psychological response to breast cancer: Effect on outcome. *Lancet* 2, 785–787.

Grossman, C. (1985). Interactions between the gonadal steroids and the immune system. *Science* 227, 257–261.

Hahn, R. C., and Petitti, D. B. (1988). Minnesota Multiphasic Personality Inventory—Rated depression and the incidence of breast cancer. *Cancer* 61, 845–848.

Ironson, G., et al. (1994). Distress, denial and low adherence to behavioral interventions predict faster disease progression in gay men infected with HIV. *International Journal of Behavioral Medicine* 1, 90–105.

Irwin, M.; Smith, T. L.; and Gillin, J. C. (1987). Low natural killer cytoxicity in major depression. *Life Sciences* 41, 2127–2133.

Kamen-Siegel, L., et al. (1991). Explanatory style and cell-mediated immunity in elderly men and women. *Health Psychology* 10, 229–235.

Kaplan, G. A., and Reynolds, P. (1988). Depression and cancer mortality and morbidity: Prospective evidence from the Alameda County study. *Journal of Behavioral Medicine* 11, 1–13.

Kemeny, M. E., and Gruenwald, T. L. (1999). Psychoneuroimmunology update. *Seminars in Gastrointestinal Disease* 10 (1), 20–29.

Knapp, P. H., et al. (1992). Short-term immunological effects of induced emotion. *Psychosomatic Medicine* 54, 133–148.

Laudenslager, M. L., et al. (1983). Coping and immunosuppression: Inescapable but not escapable shock suppresses lymphocyte proliferation. *Science* 221, 568–570.

Lin, E. H., and Peterson, C. (1990). Pessimistic explanatory style and response to illness. *Behavioral Research and Therapy* 28, 243–248.

Linn, M. W.; Linn, B. S.; and Jensen, J. (1984). Stressful events, dysphoric mood, and immune responsiveness. *Psychological Reports* 54, 219–222.

Locke, S. E., et al. (1984). Life-change stress, psychiatric symptoms, and natural killer cell activity. *Psychosomatic Medicine* 46, 441–453.

McClelland, D. C.; Alexander, C.; and Marks, E. (1980). The need for power: Stress, immune function, and illness among male prisoners. *Journal of Abnormal Psychology* 10, 93–102.

McClelland, D. C., and Krishnit, C. (1988). The effect of motivational arousal through films on salivary immunoglobulin A. *Psychology and Health* 2, 31–52.

McClelland, D. C.; Ross, G.; and Patel, V. (1985). The effect of an examination on sali-vary norepinephrine and immunoglobulin levels. *Journal of Human Stress* 11, 52–59.

Maes, M.; Bosmans, E.; Meltzer, H.; et al. (1995). Increased plasma concentrations of interleukin-6, soluble interleukin-6, soluble interleukin-2 and transferrin receptor in major depression. *Journal of Affective Disorders* 34, 301–309.

——— (1993). Interleukin-1B: A putative mediator of HPA axis hyperactivity in major depression. *American Journal of Psychiatry* 150, 1189–1193.

Maes, M.; Smith, R.; and Scharpe, S. (1995). The monocyte–T-lymphocyte hypothesis of major depression. *Psychoneuroendocrinology* 20, 111–116.

Maes, M.; Vandoolaeghe, E.; Ranjan, R.; et al. (1996). Increased serum soluble CD8 or suppressor/cytotoxic antigen concentrations in depression: Suppressive effects of glucocorticoids. *Biological Psychiatry* 40, 1273–1281.

Maier, S. F., and Watkins, L. R. (1998). Cytokines for psychologists: Implications of bidirectional immune-to-brain communication for understanding behavior, mood and cognition. *Psychological Review* 105 (1), 83–107.

Marbach, J. J.; Schleifer, S. J.; and Keller, S. E. (1990). Facial pain, distress, and immune function. *Brain Behavior and Immunity* 4, 243–254.

Morag, M., et al. (1999). Psychological variables as predictors of rubella antibody titers and fatigue—A prospective, double blind study. *Journal of Psychiatric Research* 33, 389–395.

O'Leary, A. (1990). Stress, emotion and human immune function. *Psychological Bulletin* 108, 363–382.

Pennebaker, J. W., and Beale, S. K. (1986). Confronting a traumatic event: Toward an understanding of inhibition and disease. *Journal of Abnormal Psychology* 95, 274–281.

Pennebaker, J. W.; Kiecolt-Glaser, J. K.; and Glaser, R. (1988). Disclosures of traumas and immune function: health implications for psychotherapy. *Journal of Consulting and Clinical Psychology* 56, 239–245.

Persky, V. W.; Kempthorne-Rawson, J.; and Shekelle, R. B. (1987). Personality and risk of cancer: 20-year follow-up of the Western Electric study. *Psychosomatic Medicine* 49, 435–449.

Peterson, C.; Seligman, M. E. P.; and Vaillant, G. E. (1988). Pessimistic explanatory style is a risk factor for physical illness: A 35-year longitudinal study. *Journal of Personality and Social Psychology* 55, 23–27.

Petrie, K. J.; Booth, R. J.; and Pennebaker, J. W. (1998). The immunological effects of thought suppression. *Journal of Personality and Social Psychology* 75 (5), 1264–1272.

Reed, G. M., et al. (1994). Realistic acceptance as a predictor of decreased survival time in gay men with AIDS. *Health Psychology* 13, 299–307.

Rein, G., and McRaty, R. M. (1995). Effects of positive and negative emotions on salivary IgA. *Journal of Advances in Medicine* 8, 87–105.

Reynolds, P., and Kaplan, G. A. (1990). Social connections and the risk for cancer: Prospective evidence from the Alameda County study. *Behavior Medicine* 16, 101–110.

Scheier, M. F., and Carver, C. (1992). Effects of optimism on psychological and physical well-being: Theoretical overview and empirical update. *Cognitive Therapy and Research* 16, 201–228.

Seligman, M. E. P. *Learned Optimism.* New York: Alfred Knopf, 1990.

Solomon, G. F., et al. (1987). An intensive psychoimmunologic study of long-surviving persons with AIDS: Pilot work, background studies, hypotheses, and methods. *Annals of the New York Academy of Sciences* 496, 647–655.

Stone, A. A., et al. (1987). Evidence that secretory IgA antibody is associated with daily mood. *Journal of Personality and Social Psychology* 52, 988–993.

Temoshok, L. (1985). Biopsychosocial studies on cutaneous malignant melanoma: Psycho-social factors associated with prognostic indicators, progression, psychophysiology and tumor host response. *Social Science and Medicine* 20, 833–840.

Temoshok, L. (1987). Personality, coping style, emotion and cancer: Towards an integrative model. *Cancer Surveys* 6, 545–567.

Ward, M. M., et al. (1999). Psychosocial correlates of morbidity in women with systemic lupus erythematosus. *Journal of Rheumatology* 26, 2153–2158.

Weinberger, D. A.; Schwartz, G. E.; and Davidson, R. J. (1979). Low-anxious, high-anxious, and repressive coping styles: Psychometric patterns and behavioral and physiological responses to stress. *Journal of Abnormal Psychology* 88, 369–380.

Weisse, C. S. (1992). Depression and immunocompetence: A review of the literature. *Psychological Bulletin* 111 (3), 475–489.

Wiedenfeld, S., et al. (1990). Impact of perceived self-efficacy in coping with stressors on components of the immune system. *Journal of Personality and Social Psychology* 59, 1082–1094.

Yirmiya, R. (2000). Depression in medical illness: The role of the immune system. *Western Journal of Medicine* 173, 333–336.

Chapter 3

Ader, R., and Cohen, N. (1993). Psychoneuroimmunology: Conditioning and stress. *Annual Review of Psychology* 44, 53–85.

Ader, R.; Cohen, N.; and Felten, D. (1995). Psychoneuroimmunology: Interactions between the nervous system and the immune system. *Lancet* 345, 99–103.

Antoni, M. H., et al. (1990). Psychological and neuroendocrine measures related to functional immune changes in anticipation of HIV-1 serostatus notification. *Psychosomatic Medicine* 52, 496–510.

Baron, R. S., et al. (1990). Social support and immune function among spouses of cancer patients. *Journal of Personality and Social Psychology* 59, 344–352.

Bartrop, R., et al. (1977). Depressed lymphocyte function after bereavement. *Lancet* 1, 834–836.

Benschop, R. J.; Nieuwenhuis, E.; Tromp, E.; et al. (1994). Effects of B-adrenergic blockade on immunologic and cardiovascular changes induced by mental stress. *Circulation* 89, 762–769.

Biondi, M., and Zannino, L-G. (1997). Psychological stress, neuroimmunomodulation, and susceptibility to infectious disease in animals and man. *Psychotherapy and Psychosomatics* 66 (1), 3–26.

Bovbjerg, D. H., et al. (1990). Anticipatory immune suppression and nausea in women receiving cyclic chemotherapy for ovarian cancer. *Journal of Consulting and Clinical Psychology* 58, 153–157.

Cannon, W. B. *The Wisdom of the Body.* New York: W. W. Norton, 1939.

Cohen, S., et al. (1998). Types of stressors that increase susceptibility to the common cold in healthy adults. *Health Psychology* 17, 214–223.

Cohen, S.; Tyrrell, D. A.; and Smith, A. P. (1991). Psychological stress and susceptibility to the common cold. *New England Journal of Medicine* 325, 606–612.

Fleshner, M., et al. (1989). Reduced serum antibodies associated with social defeat in rats. *Physiology and Behavior* 45, 1183–1187.

Fleshner, M., et al. (1995). RU-486 blocks differentially suppressive effect of stress on in vivo anti-KLH immunoglobulin response. *American Journal of Physiology* 271, R1344–R1352.

Glaser, J. K., et al. (1986). Modulation of cellular immunity in medical students. *Journal of Behavioral Medicine* 9, 5–21.

Green, M. L.; Green, R. G.; and Santoro, W. (1998). Daily relaxation modifies serum and salivary immunoglobulins and psychophysiologic symptom severity. *Biofeedback and Self Regulation* 13, 187–199.

Green, R. G., and Green, M. L. (1987). Relaxation increases salivary immunoglobulin A. *Psychological Reports* 61, 623–629.

Helsing, K. L.; Szklo, M.; and Comstock, E. W. (1981). Mortality after bereavement. *American Journal of Public Health* 71, 802–809.

Hewson-Bower, B., and Drummond, P. D. (1996). Secretory immunoglobulin A increases during relaxation in children with and without recurrent upper respiratory tract infection. *Journal of Developmental Behavioral Pediatrics* 17, 311–316.

Holmes, T. H., and Rahe, R. H. (1967). The social readjustment rating scale. *Journal of Psychosomatic Research* 11, 213–218.

Kiecolt-Glaser, J. K., et al. (1987). Marital quality, marital disruption, and immune function. *Psychosomatic Medicine* 49, 13–34.

Kiecolt-Glaser, J. K., et al. (1995). Slowing of wound healing by psychological stress. *Lancet* 346, 1194–1196.

Laudenslager, M. L.; Fleshner, M.; Hofstadter, P.; et al. (1988). Suppression of specific antibody production by inescapable shock: Stability under varying conditions. *Brain, Behavior, and Immunity* 2, 92–101.

Maier, S. F., and Watkins, L. R. (2000). The immune system as a sensory system: Implications for psychology. *Current Directions in Psychological Science* 9, 98–102.

Matthews, K. A., et al. (1995). Sympathetic reactivity to acute stress and immune response in women. *Psychosomatic Medicine* 57, 564–571.

McKinnon, W., et al. (1989). Chronic stress, leukocyte subpopulations, and humoral response to latent viruses. *Health Psychology* 8, 389–402.

Nakata, A.; Araki, S.; Tanigawa, T.; et al. (1996). Effect of uncontrollable and controllable electric shocks on T lymphocyte subpopulations in the peripheral blood, spleen, and thymus of rats. *Neuroimmunomodulation* 3, 336–341.

Sapolsky, R. M. (1999). Glucocorticoids, stress, and their adverse neurological effects: relevance to aging. *Experimental Gerontology* 34, 721–732.

Schleifer, S. J., et al. (1983). Suppression of lymphocyte stimulation following bereavement. *Journal of the American Medical Association* 250, 374.

Selye, H. *The Stress of Life*. New York: McGraw-Hill, 1956.

Sieber, W. J.; Rodin, J.; Larson, L.; et al. (1992). Modulation of human natural killer cell activity by exposure to uncontrollable stress. *Brain, Behavior, and Immunity* 6, 141–156.

Stone, A. A., et al. (1994). Daily events are associated with secretory immune response to an oral antigen in men. *Health Psychology* 13, 440–446.

Stone, A. A., et al. (1992). Development of common cold symptoms following experimental rhinovirus infection is related to prior stressful life events. *Behavioral Medicine* 8, 115–120.

Strauman, T. J.; Lemieux, A. M.; and Coe, C. L. (1993). Self-discrepancy and natural killer cell activity: Immunological consequences of negative self-evaluation. *Journal of Personality and Social Psychology* 64, 1042–1052.

Syvalahti, E., et al. (1985). Nonsuppression of cortisol in depression and immune function. *Neuro-Psychopharmacology and Biological Psychiatry* 9, 14–22.

Weinberger, D. A.; Schwartz, G. E.; and Davidson, R. J. (1979). Low-anxious, high-anxious, and repressive coping styles: Psychometric patterns and behavioral and physiological responses to stress. *Journal of Abnormal Psychology* 88, 369–380.

Chapter 4

Bartlett, D.; Kaufman, D.; and Smeltekop, R. (1993). The effects of music listening and perceived sensory experiences on the immune system as measured by interleukin-1 and cortisol. *Journal of Music Therapy* 30 (4), 194–209.

Blanchard, B. E. (1989). The effect of music on pulse-rate, blood pressure and final exam scores of university students. *Journal of Sports, Medicine and Physical Fitness* 19 (3), 470–471.

Blood, D., and Ferris, S. (1993). Effects of background music on anxiety, satisfaction with communication, and productivity. *Psychological Reports* 72, 171–177.

Boldt, S. (1996). The effects of music therapy on motivation, psychological well-being, physical comfort, and exercise endurance of bone marrow transplant patients. *Journal of Music Therapy* 3, 164–188.

Brennan, F. X., and Charnetski, C. J. (2000). Stress and immune system function in a newspaper's newsroom. *Psychological Reports* 87, 218–222.

Brennan, F. X.; Charnetski, C. J.; and Harrison, J. (1998). Music and Immunoglobulin A (IgA): The role of stress and affect. Paper presented at the Eastern Psychological Association annual meeting, Boston.

Brewer, J. F. (1998). Healing sounds. *Complementary Therapies in Nursing Midwifery* 4, 7–12.

Byers, J. F., and Smyth, K. A. (1997). Effect of a music intervention on noise annoyance, heart rate, and blood pressure in cardiac surgery patients. *American Journal of Critical Care* 6, 183–191.

Charnetski, C. J.; Brennan, F. X.; and Harrison, J. F. (1998). Effect of music and auditory stimuli on immunoglobulin A (IgA). *Perceptual and Motor Skills* 87, 1163–1170.

———— (1997). The effect of music on secretory immunoglobulin A (IgA). Paper presented at the Eastern Psychological Association annual meeting, Washington, D.C.

Charnetski, C. J., et al. (1989). The effect of music modality on immunoglobulin A (IgA). *Journal of the Pennsylvania Academy of Science* 63, 73–76.

Charnetski, C. J.; Timchack, S.; Peutl, N.; and Topa, J. (2001). Hemispheric priming in children with autism. Paper presented at the Eastern Psychological Association annual meeting, Washington, D.C.

Collins, S. K., and Kuck, K. (1991). Music therapy in the neonatal intensive care unit, *Neonatal Network* 99, 23–26.

Covington, H., and Crosby, C. (1997). Music therapy as a nursing intervention. *Journal of Psychosocial Nursing* 35, 34–37.

Creutzfeldt, O., and Ojemann, G. (1989). Neuronal activity in the human lateral temporal lobe III: Activity changes during music. *Experimental Brain Research* 77 (3), 490–498.

Cunningham, M. F.; Monson, B.; and Bookbinder, M. (1997). Introducing a music program in the perioperative area. *Association of Operating Room Nurses Journal* 66 (4), 674–682.

Dillon, K. M.; Minchoff, B.; and Baker, K. H. (1985). Positive emotional state and enhancement of the immune system. *International Journal of Psychiatry in Medicine* 15, 13–18.

Evans, B.; Hucklebridge, C.; and Walters, N. (1993). The relationship between secretory immunity, mood, and life events. *British Journal of Clinical Psychology* 32, 227–236.

Hanser, S. B. (1985). Music therapy and stress reduction research. *Journal of Music Therapy* 22 (4), 193–206.

Harris, C. S.; Bradley, R. J.; and Titus, S. K. (1992). A comparison of the effects of hard rock and easy-listening on the frequency of observed inappropriate behaviors: Control of environmental antecedents in a large public area. *Journal of Music Therapy* 24, 6–17.

Hicks, F. (1992). The power of music. *Nursing Times* 88, 72, 74.

Hicks, F. (1994). The role of music therapy in the care of the newborn. *Nursing Times* 91, 31–33.

Hucklebridge, F., et al. (2000). Modulation of secretory immunoglobulin A in saliva; response to manipulation of mood. *Biological Psychology* 53, 25–35.

Klein, S. A., and Winkelstein, M. L. (1997). Enhancing pediatric health care with music. *Journal of Pediatric Health Care* 10, 74–81.

Lane, D. (1992). Music Therapy: A gift beyond measure. *Oncology Nursing Society Forum* 19 (6), 863–867.

Lenton, S. R., and Martin, P. R. (1991). The contribution of music vs. instructions in the musical mood induction procedure. *Behavioral Research Therapy* 29 (6), 623–625.

McCraty, R., et al. (1996). Music enhances the effect of positive emotional states on salivary IgA. *Stress Medicine* 12, 167–175.

Monjan, A. A., and Collector, M. I. (1977). Stress-induced modulation of the immune response. *Science* 196, 307–310.

Nolan, R. S. (2000). Delta society to explore influence of animals on human health. *Journal of the American Veterans Medical Association* 21, 8–9.

Oldham, G. R., et al. (1995). Listen while you work? Quasi-experimental relations between personal-stereo headset use and employee work responses. *Journal of Applied Psychology* 80 (5), 547–564.

Rauscher, F. H.; Shaw, G. L.; and Ky, K. (1993). Music and spatial task performance. *Nature* 365, 611.

Rider, M. (1990). Imagery, improvisation, and immunity. *Psychotherapy* 17, 211–216.

Rider, M. S., et al. (1990). Effect of immune system imagery on secretory IgA. *Biofeedback Self Regulation* 15, 317–333.

Rider, M. S.; Floyd, J. W.; and Kirkpatrick, J. (1985). The effect of music therapy and relaxation on adrenal corticosteroids and the re-entrainment of circadian rhythms. *Journal of Music Therapy* 22, 46, 58.

Roberts, K. R., et al. (1998). Adolescent emotional response to music and its relationship to risk-taking behaviors. *Journal of Adolescent Health* 23, 49–54.

Routhieaux, R. L., and Tansik, D. A. (1997). The benefits of music in hospital waiting rooms. *Health Care Supervisor* 16, 31–40.

Smith, J. L., and Noon, J. (1998). Objective measurement of mood change induced by contemporary music. *Journal of Psychiatric and Mental Health Nursing* 5, 403–408.

Steckler, M. (1998). The effects of music on healing. *Journal of Long-term Home Health Care* 17 (1), 42–48.

Tobia, D. M., et al. (1999). The benefits of group music at the 1996 music weekend for women with cancer. *Journal of Cancer Education* 14, 115–119.

Updike, P. A., and Charles, D. M. (1987). Music Rx: Physiological and emotional responses to taped music programs of preoperative patients awaiting plastic surgery. *Annals of Plastic Surgery* 19, 29–33.

White, J. M. (1999). Effects of relaxing music on cardiac autonomic balance and anxiety after acute myocardial infarction. *American Journal of Critical Care* 8, 220–230.

Chapter 5

Berkman, L. S., and Syme, S. L. (1979). Social networks, host resistance, and mortality: A nine-year follow-up study of Alameda County residents. *American Journal of Epidemiology* 109, 186–204.

Charnetski, C. J., and Brennan, F. X. (1999). The effect of sexual behavior on immune function. Paper presented at the Eastern Psychological Association annual meeting, Providence, R. I.

Fahlke, C., et al. (2000). Rearing experiences and stress-induced plasma cortisol as early risk factors for excessive alcohol consumption in nonhuman primates. *Alcohol Clinical and Experimental Research* 24, 644–650.

Harlow, H. F. (1958). The nature of love. *American Psychologist* 13, 573–685.

Kiecolt-Glaser, J. K., et al. (1998). Marital stress: immunologic, neuroendocrine, and autonomic correlates. *Annals of the New York Academy of Science* 840, 656–663.

Kinsey, A. C., et al. *Sexual Behavior in the Human Female*. Philadelphia: W. B. Saunders, 1953.

Kinsey, A. C.; Pomeroy, W. B.; and Martin, C. E. *Sexual Behavior in the Human Male*. Philadelphia: W. B. Saunders, 1948.

Komisaruk, B. R., and Whipple, B. (1999). Love as sensory stimulation: Physiological consequences of its deprivation and expression. *Psychoneuroendocrinology* 23, 927–944.

Masters, W. H., and Johnson, V. E. *Human Sexual Response*. Boston: Little Brown & Company, 1964.

Ornish, D. *Love and Survival: 8 Pathways to Intimacy and Health*. New York: Harper Collins, 1998.

Pert, C. B. *Molecules of Emotion*. New York: Scribner, 1997.

Sternberg, R. J. *The Triangle of Love*. New York: Basic Books, 1988.

Strange, K. S., et al. (2000). Psychosocial stressors and mammary tumor growth: An animal model. *Neurotoxicology and Teratology* 22, 89–102.

Wedekind, C., et al. (1995). MHC-dependent mate preferences in humans. *Proceedings of the Royal Society of London and the British Biological Society* 260, 245–249.

Chapter 6

Allen, K., and Blascovich, J. (1996). The value of service dogs for people with severe ambulatory disabilities. *Journal of the American Medical Association* 75, 13, 1001–1006.

Anderson, W. P., et al. (1991). Pet ownership and risk factors for cardiovascular disease. *Medical Journal of Australia* 157, 5, 298–301.

Baun, M. M., et al. (1983). Physiological effects of human/companion animal bonding. *Nursing Research* 33, 126–129.

Brasic, J. R. (1998). Pets and health. *Psychological Reports* 83, 1011–1024.

Charnetski, C. J.; Riggers, S.; and Brennan, F. X. (2001). The effect of petting a dog on immunoglobulin A (IgA). Paper presented at the Eastern Psychological Association annual meeting, Washington, D. C.

Friedmann, E., et al. (1983). Social interaction and blood pressure: influence of animal companions. *Journal of Nervous and Mental Disease* 171, 461–465.

Friedmann, E., and Thomas, S. A. (1985). Pets and the family: Health benefits of pets for families. *Marriage and Family Review* 8, 191–203.

Holcomb, R., and Meacham, M. (1989). Effectiveness of an animal-assisted therapy program in an inpatient psychiatric unit. *Antbrozoos* 2, 259–264.

Jennings, L. B. (1997). Potential benefits of pet ownership in health promotion. *Journal of Holistic Nursing* 15, 358–372.

Jorgenson, J. (1997). Therapeutic use of companion animals in health care. *Journal of Nursing Scholarship* 29 (3), 249–254.

Lynch, J. J., et al. (1977). Human contact and cardiac arrhythmia in a coronary care unit. *Psychosomatic Medicine* 39, 188–192.

Mason, M. S., and Hagan, C. B. (1999). Pet-assisted psychotherapy. *Psychological Reports* 84, 1235–1245.

Serpell, J. (1991). Beneficial effects of pet ownership on some aspects of human health and behavior. *Journal of the Royal Society of Medicine* 84, 717–720.

Siegel, J. M. (1990). Stressful life events and use of physician services among the elderly: The moderating role of pet ownership. *Journal of Personality and Social Psychology* 58, 1081–1086.

Thomas, W. H. *Life Worth Living*. Acton, MA: VanderWyk and Burnham, 1996.

Vormbrock, J. K., and Grossberg, J. M. (1988). Cardiovascular effects of human–pet dog interactions. *Journal of Behavioral Medicine* 11, 509–517.

Winkler, A., et al. (1989). The impact of a resident dog on and institution for the elderly: Effects on perception and social interactions. *The Gerontologist* 29, 216–223.

Wright, J. C., and Moore, D. (1982). Comments on "Animal companions and one-year survival of patients after discharge." *Public Health Reports* 97, 380–381.

Yates, J. (1987). Project PUP: The perceived benefits to nursing home residents. *Antbrozoos* 1, 188–192.

Chapter 7

Berk, L. S., et al. (1989). Neuroendocrine and stress hormone changes during mirthful laughter. *American Journal of Medical Science* 298, 390–396.

Cousins, N. (1979). Anatomy of an illness (as perceived by the patient). *New England Journal of Medicine* 295, 1458–1463.

Dillon, K. M.; Minchoff, B.; and Baker, K. H. (1985). Positive emotional states and enhancement of the immune system. *International Journal of Psychiatry in Medicine* 15, 13–19.

Fry, W. F. (1992). The physiological effects of humor, mirth, and laughter. *Journal of the American Medical Association* 267, 1857–1858.

Harrison, L. K., et al. (2000). Cardiovascular and secretory immunoglobulin A reactions to humorous, exciting, and didactic film presentations. *Biological Psychology* 52, 113–126.

Labott, S. M., et al. (1990). The physiological and psychological effects on the expression and inhibition of emotion. *Behavioral Medicine* 16, 182–189.

Lambert, R. B., and Lambert, N. K. (1995). The effects of humor on secretory immunoglobulin A levels in school-aged children. *Pediatric Nursing* 21, 16–19.

Lefcourt, H. M.; Davidson-Katz, K.; and Kueneman, K. (1990). Humor and immune-system functioning. *Humor* 3, 305–321.

Martin, R. A., and Lefcourt, H. M. (1983). Sense of humor as a moderator of the relation between stressors and moods. *Journal of Personality and Social Psychology* 45, 1313–1324.

Martin, R. B.; Guthrie, C. A.; and Pitts, C. G. (1993). Emotional crying, depressed mood, and secretory immunoglobulin A. *Behavioral Medicine* 19, 111–114.

Petrie, K. J.; Booth, R. J.; and Pennebaker, J. W. (1998). The immunological effects of thought suppression. *Journal of Personality and Social Psychology* 75, 1264–1272.

Stone, A. A., et al. (1994). Daily events are associated with a secretory immune response to an oral antigen in men. *Health Psychology* 13, 440–446.

Stone, A. A., et al. (1987). Evidence that secretory IgA antibody is associated with daily mood. *Journal of Personality and Social Psychology* 5, 988–993.

Chapter 8

Ai, A. L., et al. (1998). The role of private prayer in psychological recovery among midlife and aged patients following cardiac surgery. *The Gerontologist* 38, 591–601.

Levin, J. S.; Chatters, L. M.; and Taylor, R. J. (1995). Religious effects on health status and life satisfaction among black Americans. *Journals of Gerontology—Biological Sciences, Psychological Sciences, and Social Sciences* 50, S154–S163.

Matthews, D. A. *The Faith Factor: Proof of the Healing Power of Prayer.* New York: Penguin, 1999.

McEachron, D. L., et al. (1995). Environmental lighting alters the infection process in an animal model of AIDS. *Pharmacology Biochemistry and Behavior* 51, 947–952.

Oleckno, W. A., and Blacconiere, M. J. (1991). Relationship of religiosity to wellness and other health-related behaviors and outcomes. *Psychological Reports* 68, 819–826.

Simonton, O. C.; Matthews-Simonton, S.; and Creighton, J. L. *Getting Well Again.* New York: Bantam, 1992.

Suadia, T. L., et al. (1991). Health locus of control and the helpfulness of prayer. *Heart and Lung* 20, 60–65.

Chapter 9

Ader, R., and Cohen, N. (1975). Behaviorally conditioned immunosuppression. *Psychosomatic Medicine* 37, 333–340.

———— (1982). Behaviorally conditioned immunosuppression and murine systemic lupus erythematosus. *Science* 215, 1534–1536.

Associates for Research into the Science of Enjoyment (1996). www.arise.org.

Buske-Kirschbaum, A., et al. (1992). Conditioned increase of natural killer cell activity (NKCA) in humans. *Psychosomatic Medicine* 54, 123–132.

Bybee, J. (1996). Guilt, guilt-evoking events, depression, and eating disorders. *Current Psychology* 15, 113–127.

Clow, A., et al. (1998). The effect of neutral, pleasant and unpleasant odours on salivary IgA secretion. British Psychophysiology Society meeting, London.

Hirameto, R. N., et al. (1997). Psychoneuroendocrine immunology: Site of recognition, learning and memory in the immune system and the brain. *International Journal of Neuroscience* 92 (1–2), 259–286.

Lowe, G.; Greenman, J.; and Lowe, G. (1999). Pleasure, guilt and secretory immunoglobulin A. *Psychological Reports* 85, 339–340.

Mazzeo, R. S., et al. (1998). Immune response to a single bout of exercise in young and elderly subjects. *Mechanisms of Ageing and Development* 100, 121–132.

Nieman, D. C. (1997). Exercise immunology: Practical applications. *International Journal of Sports Medicine* 18, S91–S100.

Olness, K., and Ader, R. (1992). Conditioning as an adjunct in the pharmacotherapy of lupus erythematosus. *Journal of Developmental and Behavioral Pediatrics* 13, 124–125.

Pavlov, I. P. *Conditioned Reflexes.* London: Oxford University Press, 1927.

Woods, J. A., et al. (1999). Effects of 6 months of moderate aerobic exercise training on immune function in the elderly. *Mechanisms of Ageing and Development* 109, 1–19.

Index

Underscored page references indicate boxed text.